The ICU Handbook of Facts, Formulas, and Laboratory Values

Joseph Varon, M.D.

Assistant Professor of Anesthesiology, Critical Care, and Medicine
Assistant Director, Surgical Intensive Care Unit
and Post-Anesthesia Care Unit
Assistant Director, Respiratory Care Services
The University of Texas
MD Anderson Cancer Center
Houston, Texas

Robert E. Fromm, Jr., M.D.

Associate Professor of Medicine
Sections of Cardiology, Pulmonary and Critical Care
Baylor College of Medicine
Medical Director, Emergency Services
The Methodist Hospital
Houston, Texas

Mosby

St. Louis   Baltimore   Boston
Carlsbad   Chicago   Naples   New York   Philadelphia   Portland
London   Madrid   Mexico City   Singapore   Sydney   Tokyo   Toronto   Wiesbaden

Publisher: Anne S. Patterson
Senior Editor: Laurel Craven
Developmental Editor: Kimberley Cox
Project Manager: Christopher J. Baumle
Senior Production Editor: David Orzechowski
Manufacturing Manager: William Winneberger
Cover Design: Nancy McDonald

First Edition
Copyright © 1997 by Mosby–Year Book, Inc.

Printed in the United States of America
Composition by ATLIS Graphics & Design
Printing/binding by R.R. Donnelley & Sons

Mosby–Year Book, Inc.
11830 Westline Industrial Drive
St. Louis, MO 63146

Library of Congress Cataloging in Publication Data

Varon, Joseph.
   The ICU handbook of facts, formulas, and laboratory values /
Joseph Varon, Robert E. Fromm, Jr. — 1st ed.
      p.   cm.
   Includes bibliographical references and index.
   ISBN 0-8151-8978-8
   1. Diagnosis, Differential—Tables.   2. Critical care medicine—
Tables.   3. Diagnosis, Laboratory—Tables.   I. Fromm, Robert E.
II. Title.
   [DNLM: 1. Diagnosis, Differential—handbooks.   2. Diagnosis,
Laboratory—handbooks.   3. Reference Values—handbooks.
4. Intensive Care—methods—handbooks.   WB 39 V323i 1996]
RC86.8.V365   1996
616.07′5—dc20
DNLM/DLC
for Library of Congress   96-30467
                                                                CIP

97 98 99 00 / 9 8 7 6 5 4 3 2 1

This book is dedicated to our wives (Sara and Geri), our children, and the countless students, residents, and fellows that make the ICU a challenging and exciting clinical environment year after year!

Joseph Varon, M.D.
Robert E. Fromm Jr., M.D.

Preface

The field of **Critical Care Medicine** is a relatively new one. Over the past few decades we have seen an enormous growth in the number of intensive care units (ICUs) in the United States. Thousands of medical students, residents, fellows, attending physicians, critical care nurses, pharmacists, respiratory therapists, and other health-care providers (irrespective of their ultimate field of practice) spend several months or years of their professional lives taking care of critically ill or severely injured patients. Practitioners must be able to interpret clinical data obtained by many kinds of monitoring devices, apply formulas, understand laboratory values, and then integrate this information with their knowledge of the pathophysiology of disease.

This handbook was written for everyone engaged in Critical Care Medicine. We have attempted to present basic and generally accepted clinical formulas as well as laboratory values and tables that we think should prove useful to the practitioner. In addition, formulas that help explain physiologic concepts or that underlie clinical measurements or diagnostic tests, even if not clinically useful themselves, are included. Multiple methods for deriving a particular quantity are included where appropriate. The formulas presented in the chapters of this book follow an outline format. The chapters are divided by organ system (i.e., neurologic disorders, cardiovascular disorders), as well as special topics (i.e., environmental disorders, trauma, toxicology). A special chapter outlining laboratory values is provided. In addition, each chapter reviews some formulas systematically.

Critical Care Medicine is not a static field, and changes occur every day. Therefore, this handbook is not meant to define the standard of care; but, instead, to offer a general guide to current formulas and laboratory values used in Critical Care Medicine.

Joseph Varon, M.D.
Robert E. Fromm, Jr., M.D.

Contents

Cardiovascular

Management of the critically ill requires considerable knowledge of cardiovascular performance and physiology, and how to measure these parameters. Many therapies are aimed at altering one or more cardiovascular parameters; therefore, an understanding of the relation between these variables is essential.

Accuracy in the clinical assessment of cardiovascular performance has improved importantly over the past several decades. However, an ideal method of monitoring blood flow remains to be developed. Technical difficulties with noninvasive methods have precluded their widespread adoption in the intensive care unit (ICU). Undoubtedly, further refinements and new developments will be seen in the years to come.

In the ICU, a number of guiding principles of cardiovascular care should be kept in mind:

1. **Pressure = Flow × Resistance,** this is true in the airways as well as in the cardiovascular system. For example:

Mean arterial pressure = cardiac output × systemic vascular resistance

Mean pulmonary arterial pressure = cardiac output
× pulmonary vascular resistance

The unmeasured resistance term is usually calculated by solving the equations:

$$\text{Systemic vascular resistance} = \frac{\text{mean arterial pressure}}{\text{cardiac output}}$$

2. The primary determinants of cardiovascular performance are:

Heart rate	Preload
Afterload	Contractility

3. **Other principles and conversion factors:**
   Fluid flow:

$$\text{Fluid flow} = \frac{(\text{pressure difference})(\text{radius})^4}{(\text{vessel length})(\text{fluid viscosity})^8}$$

Conversion to mm Hg:

$$\text{Pressure in mm Hg} = \text{Pressure in cm } H_2O/1.36$$

Laplace's law:

$$\text{Wall tension} = \text{distending pressure} \times \frac{\text{vessel radius}}{\text{wall thickness}}$$

Ohm's law:

$$\text{Current (I)} = \frac{\text{electromotive force (E)}}{\text{resistance (R)}}$$

Poiseuilles' law:

$$Q = v\pi r^2$$
where Q = rate of blood flow (mm/sec)
πr^2 = cross-sectional area (cm^2)
v = velocity of blood flow

Vascular capacitance:

$$\text{Vascular compliance (capacitance)} = \frac{\text{increase in volume}}{\text{increase in pressure}}$$

Vascular distensibility:

$$\text{Vascular distensibility} = \frac{\text{increase in volume}}{\text{increase in pressure} \times \text{original volume}}$$

4. Direct measurements of the heart rate are relatively easy. Preload, afterload, and contractility are more difficult to assess clinically. In assessment of cardiovascular performance, the following hemodynamic measurements are commonly measured or calculated:

Arteriovenous Oxygen Content Difference [avDO$_2$]: This is the difference between the arterial oxygen content (cao_2) and the venous oxygen content (cvo_2).

Body Surface Area (BSA): Calculated from height and weight, it is generally used to index measured and derived values according to the size of the patient.

Cardiac Index (CI): Calculated as cardiac output/BSA, it is the prime determinant of hemodynamic function.

Left Ventricular Stroke Work Index (LVSWI): It is the product of the stroke index (SI) and (mean arterial pressure [MAP] − pulmonary artery occlusion pressure [PAOP]), and a unit correction factor of 0.0136. The LVSWI measures the work of the left ventricle (LV) as it ejects into the aorta.

Mean Arterial Pressure (MAP): Estimated as one-third of pulse pressure plus the diastolic blood pressure.

Oxygen Consumption (VO$_2$): Calculated as C(a − v)O$_2$ × CO × 10, it is the amount of oxygen extracted in mL/min by the tissue from the arterial blood.

Oxygen Delivery ($\dot{D}O_2$): Calculated as (cao_2) $\times$ CO $\times$ 10, it is the total oxygen delivered by the cardiorespiratory systems.

Pulmonary Vascular Resistance Index (PVRI): Calculated as (MAP $-$ PAOP)/CI, it measures the resistance in the pulmonary vasculature.

Right Ventricular Stroke Work Index (RVSWI): It is the product of the SI and (Mean Pulmonary Artery Pressure [MPAP] $-$ Central Venous Pressure [CVP]), and a unit correction factor of 0.0136. It measures the work of the right ventricle as it ejects into the pulmonary artery.

Stroke Index (SI): Calculated as CI/heart rate, it is the average volume of blood ejected by the ventricle with each beat.

Systemic Vascular Resistance Index (SVRI): Calculated as (MAP $-$ CVP)/CI, it is the customary measure of the resistance in the systemic circuit.

Venous Admixture (Qva/Qt): Calculated as ($Cco_2 - cao_2$)/($Cco_2 - c\bar{v}o_2$), it represents the fraction of cardiac output not oxygenated in an idealized lung.

5. **Cardiac output formulas:**

$$\text{Output of left ventricle} = \frac{O_2 \text{ consumption (mL/min)}}{[cao_2 - c\bar{v}o_2]}$$

$$= \frac{250 \text{ mL/min}}{\substack{190 \text{ mL/L arterial blood} \\ - 140 \text{ mL/L venous blood} \\ \text{in pulmonary artery}}}$$

$$= \frac{250 \text{ mL/min}}{50 \text{ mL/L}} = 5 \text{ L/min}$$

It may also be measured by thermodilution techniques:

$$Q = V (Tb - Ti)K/\int Tb(t)dt$$

where

$$Q = \text{cardiac output}$$
$$V = \text{volume of injectate}$$
$$Tb = \text{blood temperature}$$
$$Ti = \text{injectate temperature}$$
$$K = \text{a constant including the density factor and catheter characteristics}$$
$$\int Tb(t)dt = \text{area under the blood-temperature-time curve}$$

These same principles are applicable for the pulmonary blood flow:

$$Q = B/(Cv - Ca)$$

where

Q = pulmonary blood flow
B = rate of loss of the indicator of alveolar gas
$C\overline{v}$ = concentration of the indicator in the venous blood
Ca = concentration of the indicator in the arterial blood

$$Q = \dot{V}O_2/(cao_2 - c\overline{v}o_2)$$

where

$\dot{Q}$ = total pulmonary blood flow
$\dot{V}O_2$ = oxygen uptake
cao_2 = arterial oxygen concentration
$c\overline{v}o_2$ = mixed venous oxygen concentration

6. **Other cardiovascular performance formulas/tables:**

Alveolar − arterial O_2 difference or "A−a gradient"
= Alveolar pO_2 − arterial pO_2

Normal < 10 torr

Alveolar pO_2 at sea level (PAo_2) = (FIO_2 × 713) − 1.2 × $Paco_2$

Arterial blood O_2 content (cao_2) = (Pao_2 × .003)
+ (1.34 × Hb in gm × arterial blood Hb O_2 sat %)

Normal = 18–20 mL/dL

Arteriovenous oxygen difference ($avDO_2$) = (cao_2) − (cvo_2)

Normal = 4–5 mL/dL

Cardiac index (CI) = cardiac output/body surface area

Normal = 3.0–3.4 L/min/m^2

Ejection Fraction (EF)
$$= \frac{\text{end-diastolic volume} - \text{end-systolic volume}}{\text{end-diastolic volume}} = \%$$

Mean arterial (or pulmonary) pressure = DBP + 1/3 (SBP- DBP)

Mean pulmonary arterial pressure = DPAP + 1/3 (SPAP − DPAP)

O_2 delivery index ($\dot{D}O_2I$) = cao_2 × cardiac index × 10

Normal = 500–600 mL/min/m^2

O_2 consumption index ($\dot{V}O_2I$) = arteriovenous O_2 difference
× cardiac index × 10

Normal = 120–160 mL/min^2

O_2 extraction (O_2 Ext) = (arteriovenous
O_2 difference/arterial blood O_2 content) × 100

Normal = 20%–30%

Pulmonary vascular resistance index (PVRI)
= 79.92 (mean PAP − PAOP)/CI

Normal = 255–285 dyne-sec/cm^5.m^2

Shunt % = (Q_s/Q_t)

$$Q_s/Q_t \ (\%) = \frac{CcO_2 - cao_2}{C_cO_2 - c\bar{v}o_2}$$

CcO_2 = Hb in gm × 1.34 + (alveolar pO$_2$ × .003)

Normal < 10%   *Considerable disease* = 20%–29%
Life-threatening > 30%

Stroke volume (SV) = (end-diastolic volume) − (end-systolic volume)

Systemic vascular resistance index (SVRI) = 79.92 (MAP − CVP/CI)

Normal = 1970 − 230 dyne-sec/cm^5.m^2

Venous blood O$_2$ content (c$\bar{v}$o$_2$) = (P$\bar{v}$O$_2$ × .003)
+ (1.34 × Hb in gm × venous blood Hb O$_2$ sat %)

Normal = 13–16 mL/dL

Table 1–1. Normal hemodynamic parameters-adult

Parameter	Equation	Normal Range
Arterial Blood Pressure (BP)	Systolic (SBP)	90–140 mm Hg
	Diastolic (DBP)	60–90 mm Hg
Mean Arterial Pressure (MAP)	[SBP + (2 × DBP)]/3	70–105 mm Hg
Right Atrial Pressure (RAP)		2–6 mm Hg
Right Ventricular Pressure (RVP)	Systolic (RVSP)	15–25 mm Hg
	Diastolic (RVDP)	0–8 mm Hg
Pulmonary Artery Pressure (PAP)	Systolic (PASP)	15–25 mm Hg
	Diastolic (PADP)	8–15 mm Hg
Mean Pulmonary Artery Pressure (MPAP)	[PASP + (2 × PADP)]/3	10–20 mm Hg
Pulmonary Artery Wedge Pressure (PAWP)		6–12 mm Hg
Left Atrial Pressure (LAP)		6–12 mm Hg
Cardiac Output (CO)	HR X SV/1000	4.0–8.0 L/min
Cardiac Index (CI)	CO/BSA	2.5–4.0 L/min/m^2
Stroke Volume (SV)	CO/HR × 1000	60–100 mL/beat
Stroke Volume Index (SVI)	CI/HR × 1000	33–47 mL/m^2/beat
Systemic Vascular Resistance (SVR)	80 × (MAP − RAP)/CO	800–1200 dynes·sec/cm^5
Systemic Vascular Resistance Index (SVRI)	80 × (MAP − RAP)/CI	1970–2390 dynes·sec/cm^5/m^2
Pulmonary Vascular Resistance (PVR)	80 × (MPAP − PAWP)/CO	<250 dynes·sec/cm^5
Pulmonary Vascular Resistance Index (PVRI)	80 × (MPAP − PAWP)/CI	255–285 dynes·sec/cm^5/m^2
Left Ventricular Stroke Work (LVSW)	SV × (MAP−PAWP) × 0.0136	58–104 gm-m/beat
Left Ventricular Stroke Work Index (LVSWI)	SVI × (MAP-PAWP) × 0.0136	50–62 gm-m/m^2/beat
Right Ventricular Stroke Work (RVSW)	SV × (MPAP-RAP) × 0.0136	8–16 gm-m/beat
Right Ventricular Stroke Work Index (RVSWI)	SV × (MPAP-RAP) × 0.0136	5–10 gm-m/m^2/beat
Coronary Artery Perfusion Pressure (CPP)	Diastolic BP-PAWP	60–80 mm Hg
Right Ventricular End-Diastolic Volume (RVEDV)	SV/EF	100–160 mL
Right Ventricular End-Systolic Volume (RVESV)	EDV-SV	50–100 mL
Right Ventricular Ejection Fraction (RVEF)	SV/EDV	40%–60%

Table 1–2. Oxygenation parameters–adult

Parameter	Equation	Normal Range
Partial Pressure of Arterial Oxygen (Pao_2)		80–100 mm Hg
Partial Pressure of Arterial CO2 ($Paco_2$)		35–45 mm Hg
Bicarbonate (HCO_3)		22–28 mEq/L
pH		7.38–7.42
Arterial Oxygen Saturation (Sao_2)		95%–100%
Mixed Venous Saturation ($S\bar{v}o_2$)		60%–80%
Arterial Oxygen Content (cao_2)	$(0.0138 \times Hb \times Sao_2) + 0.0031 \times Pao_2$	17–20 mL/dL
Venous Oxygen Content ($c\bar{v}o_2$)	$(0.0138 \times Hb \times S\bar{v}o_2) + 0.0031 \times P\bar{v}o_2$	12–15 mL/dL
A-V Oxygen Content (cao_2)	$cao_2 - c\bar{v}o_2$	4–6 mL/dL
Oxygen Delivery ($\dot{D}o_2$)	$cao_2 \times CO \times 10$	950–1150 mL/dL
Oxygen Delivery Index ($\dot{D}o_2I$)	$cao_2 \times CI \times 10$	500–600 mL/min/m^2
Oxygen Consumption ($\dot{V}o_2$)	$(C(a\text{-}\bar{v})o_2) \times CO \times 10$	200–250 mL/min
Oxygen Consumption Index ($\dot{V}o_2I$)	$(C(a\text{-}\bar{v})o_2) \times CI \times 10$	120–160 mL/min/m^2
Oxygen Extraction Ration (o_2ER)	$[(cao_2 - c\bar{v}o_2)/cao_2] \times 100$	22%–30%
Oxygen Extraction Index (o_2EI)	$(Sao_2 - S\bar{v}o_2)/Sao_2 \times 100$	25%–25%

7. **Pacemaker table:**

Table 1-3. Pacemaker classification

Letter Position	I	II	III	IV	V
	Chamber Paced	Chamber Sensed	Modes of Response	Programmable Functions	Special Antitachyarrhythmia Functions
Letters used	V–ventricle	V–ventricle	T–triggered	P–programmable (rate and/or output)	B–bursts
					N–normal rate competition
	A–atrium	A–atrium	I–inhibited	M–multiprogrammable	S–scanning
	D–double	D–double	D–double	C–communicating	
			O–none	O–none	E–external
		O–none	R–reverse		

8. **Electrocardiographic formulas/tables:**
   Rate calculation: Each large square = 0.2 seconds; 5 large squares/ second. For specific rate, measure large squares between R waves as follows:

   1 = 300 beats per minute
   2 = 150 bpm
   3 = 100 bpm
   4 = 75 bpm
   5 = 60 bpm
   6 = 50 bpm

   Axis determination: See Figs. 1–1 and 1–2.

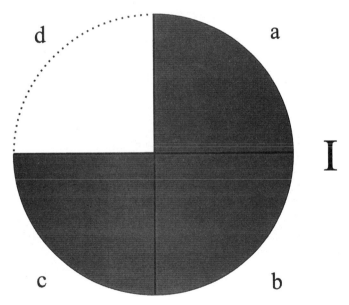

Figure 1–1.
Quadrant method for axis determination. The positive region of lead I is depicted with *vertical striping*. The positive region of aVF is shown with *horizontal striping*. By determining the orientation of lead I and aVF, the quadrant of the QRS axis can be easily determined. In quadrant *b* both lead I and aVF are positive. In quadrant *a*, lead I is positive and aVF is negative.

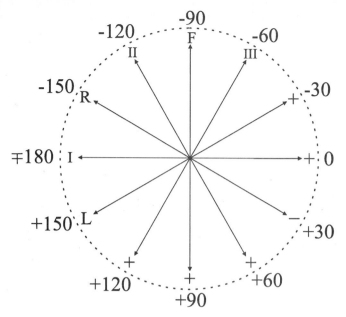

Figure 1–2.
The isoelectric method of axis determination. The location of the isoelectric lead is determined from the 12-lead ECG. The axis lies perpendicular (90°) to the isoelectric lead.

Q-T correction:

$$Q\text{-Tc} = \frac{\text{measured Q-T interval}}{\text{square root of R-R interval}}$$

9. Advanced cardiac life support (ACLS) algorithms:

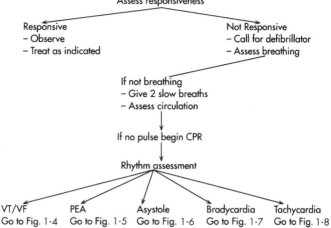

Figure 1–3.

The algorithm approach. (Modified from *JAMA* Emergency Cardiac Care Committee and Subcommittees, American Heart Association. *Guidelines for cardiopulmonary resuscitation and emergency cardiac care, III: Adult advanced cardiac life support.* 1992; 268:2216.)

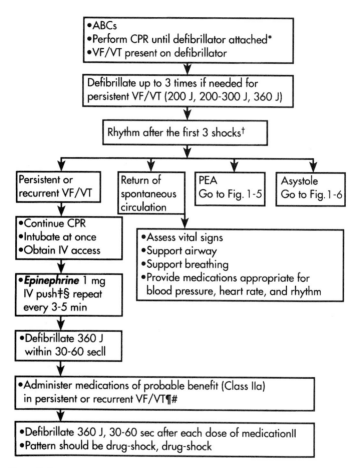

Figure 1–4

Algorithm for ventricular fibrillation (VF) and pulseless ventricular tachycardia (VT). (From *JAMA* Emergency Cardiac Care Committee and Subcommittees, American Heart Association. *Guidelines for cardiopulmonary resuscitation and emergency cardiac care, III: Adult advanced cardiac life support.* 1992; 268:2217.)

Class I: definitely helpful
Class IIa: acceptable, probably helpful
Class IIb: acceptable, possibly helpful
Class III: not indicated, may be harmful

*Precordial thump is a Class IIb action in witnessed arrest, no pulse, and no defibrillator immediately available.

†Hypothermic cardiac arrest is treated differently after this point. See section on hypothermia.

‡The recommended dose of **epinephrine** is 1 mg IV push every 3-5 min. If this approach fails, several Class IIb dosing regimens can be considered:
- Intermediate: **epinephrine** 2-5 mg IV push, every 3-5 min
- Escalating: **epinephrine** 1 mg-3 mg-5 mg IV push (3 min apart)
- High: **epinephrine** 0.1 mg/kg IV push, every 3-5 min

§**Sodium bicarbonate** (1 mEq/kg) is Class I if patient has known preexisting hyperkalemia

‖Multiple sequenced shocks (200J, 200-300J, 360J) are acceptable here (Class I), especially when medications are delayed.

¶•**Lidocaine** 1.5 mg/kg IV push. Repeat in 3-5 min to total loading dose of 3 mg/kg; then use
- **Bretylium** 5 mg/kg IV push. Repeat in 5 min at 10 mg/kg
- **Magnesium sulfate** 1-2 g IV in torsades de pointes or suspected hypomagnesemic state or severe refractory VF
- **Procainamide** 30 mg/min in refractory VF (maximum total 17 mg/kg)

#• **Sodium bicarbonate** (1 mEq/kg IV):
Class IIa
- if known preexisting bicarbonate-responsive acidosis
- if overdose with tricyclic antidepressants
- to alkalinize the urine in drug overdoses

Class IIb
- if intubated and continued long arrest interval
- upon return of spontaneous circulation after long arrest interval

Class III
- hypoxic lactic acidosis

Figure 1–4, cont'd

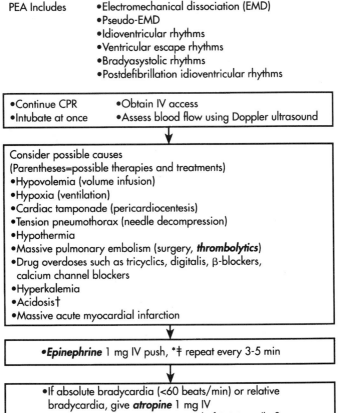

PEA Includes
- Electromechanical dissociation (EMD)
- Pseudo-EMD
- Idioventricular rhythms
- Ventricular escape rhythms
- Bradyasystolic rhythms
- Postdefibrillation idioventricular rhythms

- Continue CPR   • Obtain IV access
- Intubate at once   • Assess blood flow using Doppler ultrasound

↓

Consider possible causes
(Parentheses=possible therapies and treatments)
- Hypovolemia (volume infusion)
- Hypoxia (ventilation)
- Cardiac tamponade (pericardiocentesis)
- Tension pneumothorax (needle decompression)
- Hypothermia
- Massive pulmonary embolism (surgery, *thrombolytics*)
- Drug overdoses such as tricyclics, digitalis, β-blockers,
  calcium channel blockers
- Hyperkalemia
- Acidosis†
- Massive acute myocardial infarction

↓

- *Epinephrine* 1 mg IV push, *‡ repeat every 3-5 min

↓

- If absolute bradycardia (<60 beats/min) or relative
  bradycardia, give *atropine* 1 mg IV
- Repeat every 3-5 min up to a total of 0.04 mg/kg§

Figure 1–5.
Algorithm for pulseless electrical activity (PEA) Also known as electromechanical dissociation. (From *JAMA* Emergency Cardiac Care Committee and Subcommittees, American Heart Association. *Guidelines for cardiopulmonary resuscitation and emergency cardiac care, III: Adult advanced cardiac life support.* 1992; 268:2219.)

Class I: definitely helpful
Class IIa: acceptable, probably helpful
Class IIb: acceptable, possibly helpful
Class III: not indicated, may be harmful
*__Sodium bicarbonate__ 1mEq/kg is Class I if patient has known preexisting hyperkalemia
†__Sodium bicarbonate__ 1 mEq/kg:
  Class IIa
  • if known preexisting bicarbonate-responsive acidosis
  • if overdose with tricyclic antidepressants
  • to alkalinize the urine in drug overdoses
  Class IIb
  • if intubated and long arrest interval
  • upon return of spontaneous circulation after long arrest interval
  Class III
  • hypoxic lactic acidosis
‡The recommended dose of __epinephrine__ is 1mg IV push every 3-5 min.
If this approach fails, several Class IIb dosing regimens can be considered.
  • Intermediate: __epinephrine__ 2-5 mg IV push, every 3-5 min
  • Escalating: __epinephrine__ 1mg-3 mg-5 mg IV push (3 min apart)
  • High: __epinephrine__ 0.1mg/kg IV push, every 3-5 min
§Shorter __atropine__ dosing intervals are possibly helpful in cardiac arrest (Class IIb).

Figure 1–5, cont'd

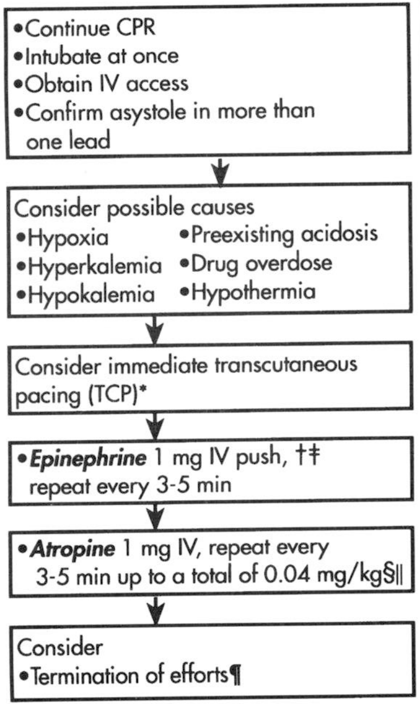

- Continue CPR
- Intubate at once
- Obtain IV access
- Confirm asystole in more than one lead

↓

Consider possible causes
- Hypoxia
- Hyperkalemia
- Hypokalemia
- Preexisting acidosis
- Drug overdose
- Hypothermia

↓

Consider immediate transcutaneous pacing (TCP)*

↓

- *Epinephrine* 1 mg IV push,†‡ repeat every 3-5 min

↓

- *Atropine* 1 mg IV, repeat every 3-5 min up to a total of 0.04 mg/kg§‖

↓

Consider
- Termination of efforts¶

Class I: definitely helpful
Class IIa: acceptable, probably helpful
Class IIb: acceptable, possibly helpful
Class III: not indicated, may be harmful

*TCP is a Class IIb intervention. Lack of success may be due to delays in pacing. To be effective TCP must be performed early, simultaneously with drugs. Evidence does not support routine use of TCP for asystole.

†The recommended dose of *epinephrine* is 1 mg IV push every 3-5 min. If this approach fails, several Class IIb dosing regimens can be considered:
- Intermediate: *epinephrine* 2-5 mg IV push, every 3-5 min
- Escalating: *epinephrine* 1 mg-3 mg-5 mg IV push (3 min apart)
- High: *epinephrine* 0.1 mg/kg IV push, every 3-5 min

‡*Sodium bicarbonate* 1 mEq/kg is Class I if patient has known preexisting hyperkalemia

§Shorter *atropine* dosing intervals are Class IIb in asystolic arrest.
‖*Sodium bicarbonate* 1 mEq/kg:
Class IIa
- if known preexisting bicarbonate-responsive acidosis
- if overdose with tricyclic antidepressants
- to alkalinize the urine in drug overdoses
Class IIb
- if intubated and continued long arrest interval
- upon return of spontaneous circulation after long arrest interval
Class III
- hypoxic lactic acidosis
¶If patient remains in asystole or other agonal rhythms after successful intubation and initial medications and no reversible causes are identified, consider termination of resuscitative efforts by a physician. Consider interval since arrest.

Figure 1-6.
Asystole treatment algorithm. (From *JAMA* Emergency Cardiac Care Committee and Subcommittees, American Heart Association. *Guidelines for cardiopulmonary resuscitation and emergency cardiac care, III: Adult advanced cardiac life support.* 1992; 268:2220.)

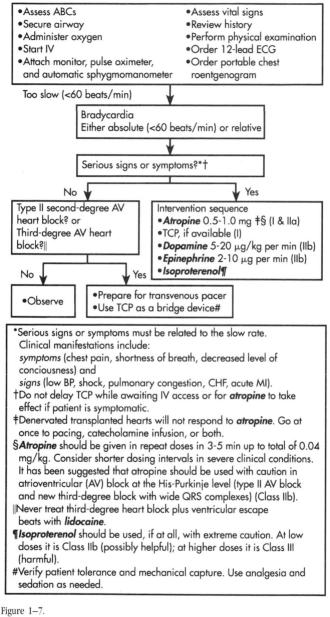

• Assess ABCs	• Assess vital signs
• Secure airway	• Review history
• Administer oxygen	• Perform physical examination
• Start IV	• Order 12-lead ECG
• Attach monitor, pulse oximeter, and automatic sphygmomanometer	• Order portable chest roentgenogram

Too slow (<60 beats/min)

Bradycardia
Either absolute (<60 beats/min) or relative

Serious signs or symptoms?*†

No

Type II second-degree AV heart block? or
Third-degree AV heart block?‖

No | **Yes**

• Observe

• Prepare for transvenous pacer
• Use TCP as a bridge device#

Yes

Intervention sequence
• *Atropine* 0.5-1.0 mg ‡§ (I & IIa)
• TCP, if available (I)
• *Dopamine* 5-20 μg/kg per min (IIb)
• *Epinephrine* 2-10 μg per min (IIb)
• *Isoproterenol*¶

*Serious signs or symptoms must be related to the slow rate.
  Clinical manifestations include:
  symptoms (chest pain, shortness of breath, decreased level of conciousness) and
  signs (low BP, shock, pulmonary congestion, CHF, acute MI).
†Do not delay TCP while awaiting IV access or for *atropine* to take effect if patient is symptomatic.
‡Denervated transplanted hearts will not respond to *atropine*. Go at once to pacing, catecholamine infusion, or both.
§*Atropine* should be given in repeat doses in 3-5 min up to total of 0.04 mg/kg. Consider shorter dosing intervals in severe clinical conditions. It has been suggested that atropine should be used with caution in atrioventricular (AV) block at the His-Purkinje level (type II AV block and new third-degree block with wide QRS complexes) (Class IIb).
‖Never treat third-degree heart block plus ventricular escape beats with *lidocaine*.
¶*Isoproterenol* should be used, if at all, with extreme caution. At low doses it is Class IIb (possibly helpful); at higher doses it is Class III (harmful).
#Verify patient tolerance and mechanical capture. Use analgesia and sedation as needed.

Figure 1–7.
Bradycardia treatment algorithm. (From *JAMA* Emergency Cardiac Care Committee and Subcommittees, American Heart Association. *Guidelines for cardiopulmonary resuscitation and emergency cardiac care, III: Adult advanced cardiac life support.* 1992; 268:2221.)

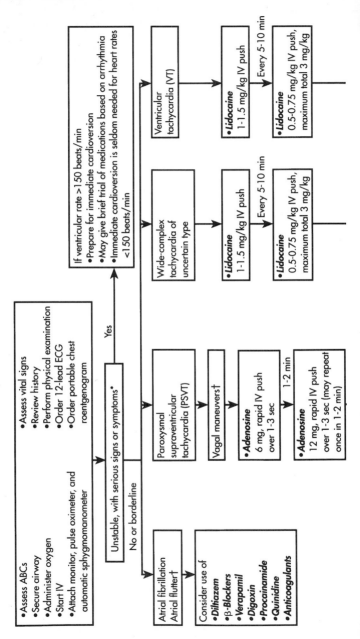

- Assess ABCs
- Secure airway
- Administer oxygen
- Start IV
- Attach monitor, pulse oximeter, and automatic sphygmomanometer

- Assess vital signs
- Review history
- Perform physical examination
- Order 12-lead ECG
- Order portable chest roentgenogram

Unstable, with serious signs or symptoms*

No or borderline

Yes

If ventricular rate >150 beats/min
- Prepare for immediate cardioversion
- May give brief trial of medications based on arrhythmia
- Immediate cardioversion is seldom needed for heart rates <150 beats/min

Atrial fibrillation
Atrial flutter†

Consider use of
- *Diltiazem*
- *β-Blockers*
- *Verapamil*
- *Digoxin*
- *Procainamide*
- *Quinidine*
- *Anticoagulants*

Paroxysmal supraventricular tachycardia (PSVT)

Vagal maneuvers†

- *Adenosine*
  6 mg, rapid IV push over 1-3 sec

1-2 min

- *Adenosine*
  12 mg, rapid IV push over 1-3 sec (may repeat once in 1-2 min)

Wide-complex tachycardia of uncertain type

- *Lidocaine*
  1-1.5 mg/kg IV push

Every 5-10 min

- *Lidocaine*
  0.5-0.75 mg/kg IV push, maximum total 3 mg/kg

Ventricular tachycardia (VT)

- *Lidocaine*
  1-1.5 mg/kg IV push

Every 5-10 min

- *Lidocaine*
  0.5-0.75 mg/kg IV push, maximum total 3 mg/kg

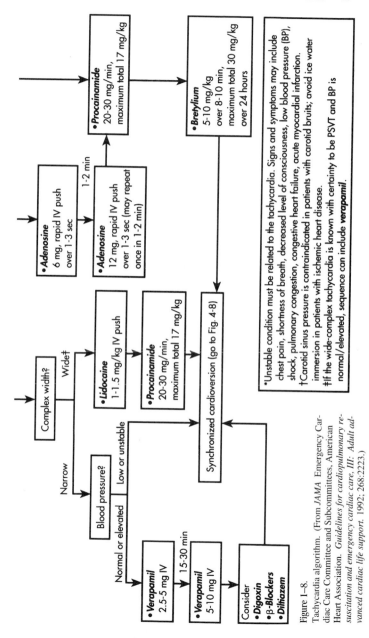

Figure 1–8.
Tachycardia algorithm. (From *JAMA* Emergency Cardiac Care Committee and Subcommittees. American Heart Association. *Guidelines for cardiopulmonary resuscitation and emergency cardiac care, III: Adult advanced cardiac life support.* 1992; 268:2223.)

Complex width?

Narrow

Blood pressure?

Normal or elevated

•*Verapamil*
2.5–5 mg IV

15–30 min

•*Verapamil*
5–10 mg IV

Consider
•*Digoxin*
•*β-Blockers*
•*Diltiazem*

Low or unstable

Wide‡

•*Lidocaine*
1–1.5 mg/kg IV push

•*Procainamide*
20–30 mg/min,
maximum total 17 mg/kg

Synchronized cardioversion (go to Fig. 4-8)

•*Adenosine*
6 mg, rapid IV push
over 1–3 sec

•*Adenosine*
12 mg, rapid IV push
over 1–3 sec (may repeat
once in 1–2 min)

1–2 min

•*Procainamide*
20–30 mg/min,
maximum total 17 mg/kg

•*Bretylium*
5–10 mg/kg
over 8–10 min,
maximum total 30 mg/kg
over 24 hours

*Unstable condition must be related to the tachycardia. Signs and symptoms may include chest pain, shortness of breath, decreased level of consciousness, low blood pressure (BP), shock, pulmonary congestion, congestive heart failure, acute myocardial infarction.

†Carotid sinus pressure is contraindicated in patients with carotid bruits; avoid ice water immersion in patients with ischemic heart disease.

‡If the wide-complex tachycardia is known with certainty to be PSVT and BP is normal/elevated, sequence can include *verapamil*.

Tachycardia with serious signs and symptoms related to the tachycardia

If ventricular rate is >150 beats/min, prepare for immediate cardioversion.
May give brief trial of medications based on specific arrhythmias.
Immediate cardioversion is generally not needed for rates <150 beats/min.

Check
•Oxygen saturation   •IV line
•Suction device   •Intubation equipment

Premedicate whenever possible*

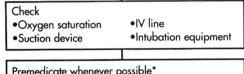

Synchronized cardioversion†‡
VT§
PSVT‖
Atrial fibrillation   — 100 J, 200 J, 300 J, 360 J‡
Atrial flutter‖

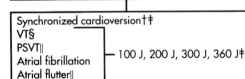

*Effective regimens have included a sedative (eg, *diazepam, mida-zolam, barbiturates, ethomidate, ketamine, methohexital*) with or without an analgesic agent (eg, *fentanyl, morphine, meperidine*). Many experts recommend anesthesia if service is readily available.
†Note possible need to resynchronize after each cardioversion.
‡If delays in synchronization occur and clinical conditions are critical, go to immediate unsynchronized shocks.
§Treat polymorphic VT (irregular form and rate) like VF: 200 J, 200-300 J, 360 J.
‖PSVT and atrial flutter often respond to lower energy levels (start with 50 J).

Figure 1–9.
Electrical cardioversion algorithm (with the patient not in cardiac arrest). (From *JAMA* Emergency Cardiac Care Committee and Subcommittees, American Heart Association. *Guidelines for cardiopulmonary resuscitation and emergency cardiac care, III: Adult advanced cardiac life support.* 1992; 268:2224.)

10. Common dysrhythmias

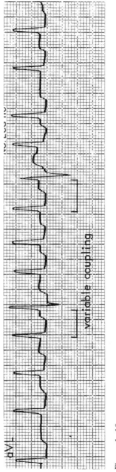

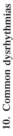

Figure 1–10.
Atrial fibrillation. (From Varon J, ed: *Practical Guide to the Care of the Critically Ill Patient.* St. Louis, Mosby–Year Book, Inc., 1994:393–398.)

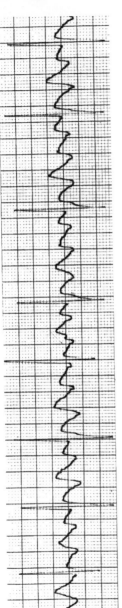

Figure 1–11.
Atrial flutter. (From Varon J, ed: *Practical Guide to the Care of the Critically Ill Patient.* St. Louis, Mosby–Year Book, Inc., 1994:393–398.)

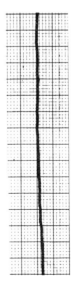

Figure 1–12.
Asystole. (From Varon J, ed: *Practical Guide to the Care of the Critically Ill Patient.* St. Louis, Mosby–Year Book, Inc., 1994: 393–398.)

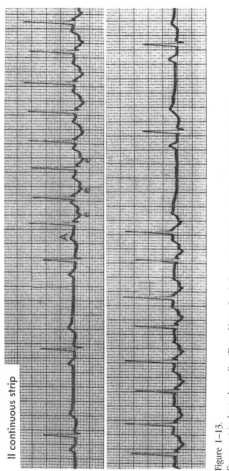

Figure 1–13.
Supraventricular tachycardia. (From Varon J, ed: *Practical Guide to the Care of the Critically Ill Patient*. St. Louis, Mosby–Year Book, Inc., 1994:393–398.)

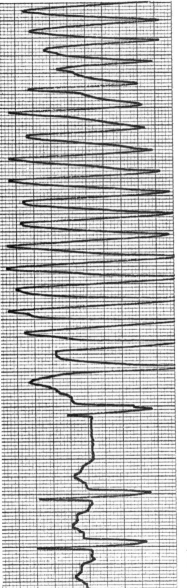

Figure 1–14.
Torsades de pointes. (From Varon J, ed: *Practical Guide to the Care of the Critically Ill Patient.* St. Louis, Mosby–Year Book, Inc., 1994:393–398.)

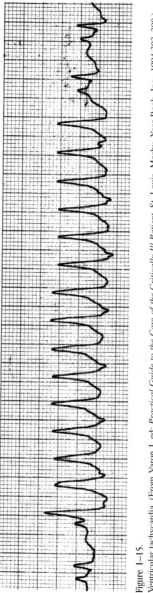

Figure 1–15.
Ventricular tachycardia. (From Varon J, ed: *Practical Guide to the Care of the Critically Ill Patient.* St. Louis, Mosby–Year Book, Inc., 1994:393–398.)

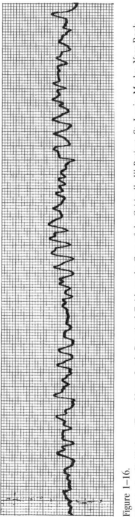

Figure 1–16.
Ventricular fibrillation. (From Varon J, ed: *Practical Guide to the Care of the Critically Ill Patient*. St. Louis, Mosby–Year Book, Inc., 1994:393–398.)

Endocrinology and Metabolism

Alterations in endocrine function and metabolism are common in critically ill patients. Laboratory testing and interpretation of laboratory data plays an important part in the management of these disorders.

1. **Adrenal function:** The question of adrenal insufficiency in critically ill patients arises commonly.

   Serum cortisol ≥ 20 μg/dL = adequate adrenal function

Formal *ACTH stimulation test* (may be measured while administering dexamethasone 10 mg IV q 6 h):

- Baseline cortisol
- 0.25 mg cosyntropin IV
- Cortisol level at 60 min
- < 7 μg/dL increase suggests primary adrenal insufficiency if basal is < 20 mcg/dL

Corticosteroids are commonly used in inflammatory disorders and for replacement therapy. Equivalent doses are listed in Table 2–1.

Table 2–1. Equivalent corticosteroid doses

| Agent | Dose (mg) | Duration | Potency | |
			Mineralocorticoid	Glucocorticoid
Cortisol	20.0	8h	1.0	1.0
Cortisone	25.0	8h	1.0	0.8
Dexamethasone	0.75	72h	0	25
Hydrocortisone	25.0	8h	1.0	0.8
Methylprednisolone	4.0	36h	0.5	5
Prednisolone	5.0	24h	0.8	4
Prednisone	5.0	24h	0.8	4

2. **Diabetes insipidus (DI):** A disorder of fluid homeostasis caused by inadequate antidiuretic hormone (ADH) secretion or action:

Neurogenic DI = Inadequate production or secretion of ADH

Nephrogenic DI = Unresponsiveness of renal tubules to ADH

The *water deprivation test* may be performed if the patient is hemodynamically stable and the serum sodium is <145 mEq/L (Table 2–2).

3. **Sodium formulas:**
   Serum sodium correction in hyperglycemia:
   $$Na^+_{euglycemic} = \text{measured } Na^+ + 0.028 \text{ (glucose } - 100)$$

   Serum sodium correction in hyperlipidemia and hyperproteinemia:

   decrease (mEq/L) serum Na^+ in hyperlipidemia
   = plasma lipids (mg/dL) × 0.002

   decrease (mEq/L) serum Na^+ in hyperproteinemia
   = increment of total protein >8 g/dL × 0.25

   Estimated sodium excess in hypernatremia:

   Na^+ excess (mEq/L) = 0.6 body weight (Kg)
   × (current plasma Na^+ − 140)

   Estimated sodium deficit in hyponatremia:

   Na^+ deficit (mEq) = 0.6 × body weight × (desired
   plasma Na^+ − current plasma Na^+)

4. **Osmolality formulas:**

   $$\text{Calculated osmolality} = 2\,(Na^+ + K^+) + \frac{\text{Glucose}}{18} + \frac{\text{BUN}}{2.8}$$

   $$\text{Effective osmolality} = 2\,(Na^+) + \frac{\text{Glucose}}{18}$$

   Osmolal gap = Measured osmolality − calculated osmolality

Table 2–2. Water deprivation test

	Maximum Uosm (mOsm/kg H₂O)	Maximum Uosm / Posm	% change after vasopressin*	Maximum Uosm/Posm after vasopressin*
Normal	800–1200	>1	<9	>1
Partial diabetes insipidus	400	>1	>9	>1
Complete diabetes insipidus	100–200	<1	>50	variable
Nephrogenic diabetes insipidus	<150	<1	<45	<1

*5 U subcutaneously

5. **Diabetes mellitus:** Complications of diabetes mellitus may be the presenting condition of a patient in the ICU. However, many other patients may develop glucose intolerance while in the ICU. Diabetic ketoacidosis (DKA) and nonketotic hyperosmolar coma (HNKC) may present similarly. The characteristics listed in Tables 2–3 and 2–4 may help the clinician differentiate between the two.

Table 2–3. Laboratory presentation of DKA and HNKC

Laboratory test	DKA	HNKC
Blood glucose (mg/dL)	200–2000	usually >600
Blood ketones	present	absent
Arterial pH	<7.4	normal*
Anion gap	↑↑	normal or ↑↑
Osmolality	↑	↑↑
Urine dipstick	glucose and ketones	glucose

DKA = diabetic ketoacidosis, HNKC = Hyperglycemic non-ketotic coma, ↑ = slightly elevated, ↑↑ = elevated
*May be low if hypovolemia causes poor tissue perfusion

Table 2–4 contains some of the insulins commonly employed in the ICU setting

Table 2–4. Types of insulins commonly employed in the ICU

Type of insulin	Onset of action	Peak	Duration
Regular (IV)	5 minutes	20–25 minutes	40–45 minutes
Regular (IM)	30 minutes	60 minutes	90–100 minutes
Regular (SQ)	60 minutes	180 minutes	360 minutes
NPH (SQ)	240 minutes	360–480 minutes	600–960 minutes
Lente (SQ)	240 minutes	360–480 minutes	600–960 minutes
Ultralente (SQ)	480–720 minutes	720–1080 minutes	1080–1680 minutes

6. Hypoglycemia (Table 2–5)

Table 2–5. Differentiating exogenous insulin administration, insulinoma, and oral hypoglycemic agents-induced hypoglycemia. Other causes of hypoglycemia such as hepatic failure should be considered in the ICU

Laboratory test	Insulinoma	Exogenous insulin	Sulfonylureas
Plasma insulin level	↑	↑↑	↑
Insulin antibodies	None*	Present	None*
Plasma/urine sulfonylurea levels	Absent	Absent	Present
C-peptide	↑	N/↓	↑

*May be present if the patient has had prior insulin injections.
↑↑ = increased, ↓ = decreased, N = normal

7. Thyroid function tests (Tables 2–6 and 2–7).

Table 2–6. Thyroid function tests

Direct methods	Indirect methods
Circulating levels of total hormones	*Thyroid hormone binding test*
total thyroxine (T_4)	resin uptake of $^{125}I\text{-}T_3$
total triiodothyronine (T_3)	
protein bound iodine (PBI)	
Circulating levels of free hormones	Free thyroxine index (FTI)
free thyroxine (fT_4)	$$FTI = \frac{T_4 \times \text{patient triiodothyronine } (T_3)}{\text{control triiodothyronine } (T_3)}$$
free triiodothyronine (fT_3)	
Thyroid hormone binding proteins	
thyroxine binding globulin (TBG)	

Table 2–7. Interpretation of thyroid function tests in the ICU

Test	Hypothyroid	High T_4 syndrome	Hyperthyroid	Low T_3 syndrome	Low T_3/T_4 syndrome
TSH	high*	Nl/low	low	low to sl ↑	low to sl ↑
Total T_4	low	high	high	Nl	low
Total T_3	low to low Nl	low/Nl/high	high	low	low
Reverse T_3	Nl/low	Nl/high	high	high	high
Free T_4	low	Nl/high	high	Nl	Nl
T_3RU	low	Nl/low	high	Nl/high	high

Nl = normal; sl = slight

* = except TSH is low in hypothyroidism of secondary and tertiary causes

8. Calcium metabolism and disorders:

$$\text{Corrected } Ca^{++} = \text{Measured } Ca^{++} + 0.8 \times (4 - \text{plasma albumin})$$

$$\text{Corrected } Ca^{++} \text{ (quick method)} = Ca^{++} - \text{albumin} + 4$$

In the differential diagnosis of hypercalcemia the use of urinary cyclic AMP and parathyroid hormone may confirm a diagnosis (Table 2–8).

Table 2–8. Use of iPTH and urinary cyclic AMP in the differential diagnosis of hypercalcemia

iPTH	Urinary cyclic AMP	iPLP	Diagnosis
↑↑	↑↑	N	Primary hyperparathyroidism
N or ↓	N or ↓	↑	Probable occult malignancy

↑ = increased, ↓ = decreased, N = normal
iPTH = Parathyroid hormone by radioimmunoassay; iPLP = parathyroid hormone-like protein by radioimmunoassay.

9. Nutrition formulas:
Please refer to Chapter 8 for additional formulas. The *body mass index* (BMI) is frequently utilized when dealing with nutrition in the critically ill patient:

$$\text{BMI} = \frac{\text{(Body weight [Kg])}}{\text{(Height [m])}^2}$$

Harris-Benedict equation: It measures the basal energy expenditure (BEE) which represents the resting basal metabolic rate:

Men:

$$66 + (13.7 \times W) + (\% \times H) - (6.8 \times A) = \text{kcal/day}$$

Women:

$$655 + (9.6 \times W) + (1.7 \times H) - (4.7 \times A) = \text{kcal/day}$$

where W = body weight in kilograms, H = height in centimeters, and A = age in years

Nitrogen balance (NB): Requires knowledge of protein intake urine urea nitrogen (UUN). For patients with normal renal function the following formula is utilized:

$$\text{NB} = (\text{Dietary protein} \times 0.16) - (\text{UUN} + 2 \text{ g stool} + 2 \text{ g skin})$$

In patients with renal dysfunction, the increased blood urea pool and extrarenal losses must be accounted for, and the following formula is used:

$$\text{NB} = \text{Nitrogen in} - (\text{UUN} + 2 \text{ g stool} + 2 \text{ g skin} + \text{BUN change})$$

The *catabolic index* (CI) is derived from the same variables:

$$\text{CI} = \text{UUN} - [(0.5 \times \text{dietary protein} \times 0.16) + 3 \text{ g}]$$

Environment

Physical factors such as temperature, pressure, altitude, and humidity affect gases in particular and thus should be well understood by the critical care practitioner. A number of useful tables, formulas, and figures follow. Thermal injuries are commonly considered environmental events, and formulas and figures concerning them are included in this chapter.

1. **Temperature:** Temperature conversions are often calculated during the management of critically ill patients. Degrees *Celsius* (°C) and *Fahrenheit* (°F) are the most commonly converted.
   °C to °F

   $$°F = (°C \times 9/5) + 32$$

   °F to °C

   $$°C = (°F - 32) \times 5/9$$

Occasionally, the *Kelvin* (K) temperature scale is used, particularly in gas law calculations:
K to °C

$$K = °C + 273$$

2. **Humidity:** *Relative humidity* (RH) is usually measured by hygrometers; thus, eliminating the need of extracting and measuring the humidity content of the air samples:

$$RH = \frac{\text{Content [mg/L or mm Hg]}}{\text{Capacity [mg/L or mm Hg]}} = \%$$

The *humidity deficit* (HD) represents the maximum humidity capacity at body temperature:

$$HD = \text{Capacity} - \text{content} = mg/L$$

where *capacity* represents the amount of water the alveolar air can hold at body temperature (also known as absolute humidity) and *content* represents the humidity content of inspired air (Table 3–1).

Table 3–1. Humidity capacity of saturated gases from 0–43 °C

Gas temperature (°C)	Water content (mg/L)	Water vapor pressure (mm Hg)
0	4.9	4.6
5	6.8	6.6
10	9.4	9.3
17	14.5	14.6
18	15.4	15.6
19	16.3	16.5
20	17.3	17.5
21	18.4	18.7
22	19.4	19.8
23	20.6	21.1
24	21.8	22.4
25	23.1	23.8
26	24.4	25.2
27	25.8	26.7
28	27.2	28.3
29	28.8	30.0
30	30.4	31.8
31	32.0	33.7
32	33.8	35.7
33	35.6	37.7
34	37.6	39.9
35	39.6	42.2
36	41.7	44.6
37	43.9	47.0
38	46.2	49.8
39	48.6	52.5
40	51.1	55.4
41	53.7	58.4
42	56.5	61.6

3. **Pressure:** *Pressure* is defined as force per unit area, and there are various ways of measuring this force. One way is that force can be recorded in a form of the height of a column, as in the mercury barometer; therefore, it can be recorded in millimeters of mercury (mm Hg) pressure or centimeters of water pressure. To convert *cm H_2O to mm Hg*:

$$\text{cm } H_2O \times 0.735 = \text{mm Hg}$$

To convert *mm Hg* to *cm H_2O*:

$$\text{mm Hg} \times 1.36 = \text{cm } H_2O$$

A less commonly used conversion in clinical medicine includes converting *psi* to *mm Hg*:

$$\text{Psi} \times 51.7 = \text{mm Hg}$$

Other useful pressure-related formulas/facts include:

$$\text{Total pressure} = P_1 + P_2 + P_3 + \ldots\ (\textit{Dalton's law})$$

$$
\begin{aligned}
1\ \text{atmosphere} &= 760\ \text{mm Hg} \\
&= 29.921\ \text{in Hg} \\
&= 33.93\ \text{ft } H_2O \\
&= 1034\ \text{cm } H_2O \\
&= 1034\ \text{gm/cm}^2 \\
&= 14.7\ \text{lb/in}^2
\end{aligned}
$$

Useful pressure/volume relationships that can be used in the management of critically ill patients include:

$$\text{Volume}_{BTPS} = \text{Volume}_{ATPS} \times \text{Factor}$$

where *Volume$_{BTPS}$* is the gas volume saturated with water at body temperature (37°C) and ambient pressure [BTPS = barometric temperature pressure saturation]; *Volume$_{ATPS}$* is the gas volume saturated with water at ambient (room) temperature and pressure [ATPS = ambient temperature pressure saturation]; *Factor* represents the factors for converting gas volumes from ATPS to BTPS (Table 3–2):

$$\text{Conversion factor} = \frac{P_B - PH_2O}{P_B - 47} \times \frac{310}{(273 + °C)}$$

Table 3–2. Factors for converting gas volumes from ATPS to BTPS

Gas temperature (°C)	Factors to convert to 37°C saturated	Water vapor pressure (mm Hg)
18	1.112	15.6
19	1.107	16.5
20	1.102	17.5
21	1.096	18.7
22	1.091	19.8
23	1.085	21.1
24	1.080	22.4
25	1.075	23.8
26	1.068	25.2
27	1.063	26.7
28	1.057	28.3
29	1.051	30.0
30	1.045	31.8
31	1.039	33.7
32	1.032	35.7
33	1.026	37.7
34	1.020	39.9
35	1.014	42.2
36	1.007	44.6
37	1.000	47.0
38	0.993	49.8
39	0.986	52.5
40	0.979	55.4
41	0.971	58.4
42	0.964	61.6

4. Altitude: As altitude varies, changes in atmospheric pressure produce alterations in gas density (Table 3–3).

Table 3–3. Changes in density with altitude assuming a constant temperature

Altitude (Feet)	Standard temperature (°C)	Density ratio Constant temperature	Density ratio Standard temperature
0	15.00	1.0000	1.0000
5000	5.09	0.8320	0.8617
10000	−4.81	0.6877	0.7385
15000	−14.72	0.5643	0.6292

5. **Burns:** To estimate the extent of burn, the *rule of nines* for body surface area (BSA) is commonly used:

Adults: arms 9 percent each; legs 18 percent each; head 9 percent; trunk 18 percent anterior, 18 percent posterior; genitalia 1 percent.

Children: arms 9 percent each; legs 16 percent each; head 13 percent; trunk 18 percent anterior, 18 percent posterior; genitalia 1 percent.

Infants: arms 9 percent each; legs 14 percent each; head 18 percent; trunk 18 percent anterior, 18 percent posterior; genitalia 1 percent.

In addition, the *Lund and Browder chart* (Fig. 3–1) can be used (more accurate in children):

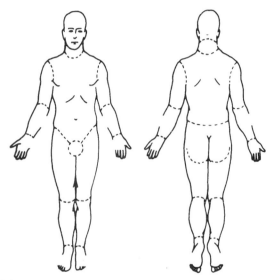

Figure 3–1
Lund and Browder chart for estimation of burn extent. (From Artz CP and Yarbrough DR III: *Burns: including cold, chemical, and electrical injuries.* In Sabiston CC, Jr, editor: *Textbook of surgery: the biological basis of modern surgical practice,* ed 11, Philadelphia, 1977, WB Saunders.)

Gastroenterology

Disorders of the gastrointestinal (GI) system commonly result in ICU admissions. In addition, critically ill patients may suffer stress-induced mucosal injury, ileus, and hepatic dysfunction. The following formulas and facts should be useful in a broad range of ICU patients. Many additional important facts and formulas related to the GI tract can be found in Chapter 8 (Nutrition).

1. **Intestinal transit:** The normal 24-hour *intestinal fluid* and *electrolyte transport* is depicted in Table 4–1:

Table 4–1. Normal 24-hour intestinal fluid and electrolyte transport

Site	Fluid received (L)	Amount absorbed (L)	Electrolyte absorption		
			Na^+	K^+	Cl^-
Duodenum/ jejunum	9.0	4.0	Passive	Passive	Passive
Ileum	5.0	3.5	Active	Passive	Passive
Colon	1.5	1.35	Active	Passive	Active

2. **Stool formulas:** As part of the diagnostic work-up of patients with diarrhea, *stool osmolal gap* (SOG) is usually calculated by the following formula:

$$SOG = \text{stool osmolality} - 2 \times (\text{stool } Na^+ + \text{stool } K^+)$$

Normal stool osmolality is <290 mOsm/L. If the SOG >100 it indicates an osmotic diarrhea.

3. Liver facts: The *Child's classification* for portal hypertension is commonly used in critically ill patients and is depicted in Table 4–2:

Table 4–2. Child's classification of portal hypertension

Class	A	B	C
Serum bilirubin (mg/dL)	<2	2–3	>3
Serum albumin (g/dL)	>3.5	3–5	<3
Ascites	None	Easily controlled	Poorly controlled
Encephalopathy	None	Minimal	Advanced
Nutrition	Excellent	Good	Poor

4. Hepatitis:

The interpretation of laboratory tests performed in patients with *viral hepatitis* is depicted in Table 4–3.

Table 4–3. Interpretation of hepatitis profiles

IgM Anti-HAV	HBsAg	IgM Anti-HBc	Anti-HBs	HBeAg	Anti-HBe	Anti-HDV	Interpretation
−	−	−	−	−	−	−	Clinical acute hepatitis may be caused by non-A, non-B hepatitis, other viral infection, or liver toxin
+	−	−	−	−	−	−	Acute type A hepatitis
−	+	+	−	+	−	−	Late incubation period or early acute type B hepatitis
−	+	+	−	+	−	−	Acute type B hepatitis with persistent viral replication (HB$_s$Ag+) and high degree of infectivity (HB$_e$Ag+)
−	+	+	−	−	+	−	Acute type B hepatitis with favorable prognosis for resolution (seroconversion of HB$_e$Ag to anti-HB$_e$)
−	−	+	−	−	−/+	−	Acute infection nearly resolved (core window)
−	−	+/−	+	−	−/+	−	Convalescent phase of type B hepatitis with recovery and immunity
−	−	−	+	−	−	−	Past type B hepatitis long before with recovery and immunity, passive transfer of antibody (HBIG), or hepatitis B vaccine
−	+	+	−	+/−	−	+	Acute hepatitis B with acute hepatitis delta coinfection
−	+	−	−	−	−	+	Chronic hepatitis B with acute hepatitis delta superinfection
−	+	−	−	−	−	++	Chronic hepatitis B with chronic delta hepatitis

Modified from Sass MA, Cianflocco AJ: Resid Staff Physician 34(4):17PC, 1985.

Hematology

Patients in the intensive care unit frequently have hematologic problems. These include anemia, coagulopathies, and thrombocytosis, to name just a few. In evaluating these patients, many laboratory tests and indices are obtained. The following formulas will aid the critical care practitioner in evaluating hematologic parameters.

1. **Red blood cells:** The *mean corpuscular volume* (MCV) indicates the average volume of a single RBC in a given blood sample and is calculated as:

$$MCV = \frac{Hct\ (\%) \times 10}{RBC\ (10^{12}/L)}$$

The *mean corpuscular hemoglobin* (MCH) indicates the average weight of Hb per erythrocyte:

$$MCH = \frac{Hb\ (g/dL) \times 10}{RBC\ (10^{12}/L)}$$

The *mean corpuscular hemoglobin concentration* (MCHC) indicates the average concentration of Hb in the RBCs of any specimen:

$$MCHC = \frac{Hb\ (g/dL)}{Hct\ (\%)} \times 100$$

The *red blood cell volume* can be calculated via a radionuclide study:

$$RBC\ volume = \frac{cpm\ of\ isotope\ injected}{cpm/mL\ RBC\ in\ sample}$$

where cpm = counts per million

2. **Reticulocytes counts:** To calculate the *percentage* of *retriculocytes*, usually based on counting 1000 RBCs, the following formula is commonly utilized:

$$Reticulocytes\ (\%) = \frac{Number\ of\ reticulocytes}{Number\ of\ RBC\ observed} \times 100$$

The *actual reticulocyte count* (ARC) reflects the actual number of reticulocytes in one liter of whole blood:

$$ARC = \frac{\text{Reticulocytes (\%)}}{100} \times RBC \text{ count } (\times 10^{12}/L) \times 1000$$

The corrected reticulocyte count (CRC) is calculated as:

$$CRC = \text{Reticulocytes (\%)} \times \frac{Hct \text{ (L/L)}}{0.45 \text{ L/L}}$$

The reticulocyte count is usually viewed in relation to the degree of anemia. The *reticulocyte production index* (RPI) is a frequently used correction method:

$$RPI = \frac{(\text{Measured Hct/Normal Hct}) \times \text{Reticulocyte count}}{\text{Maturation time in peripheral blood}}$$

The *maturation factor* varies according to the hematocrit in the following manner (Table 5–1).

Table 5–1. Maturation of reticulocytes in peripheral blood

Hematocrit	Maturation time in days
0.41–0.50	1
0.30–0.40	1.5
0.20–0.39	2
0.10–0.19	2.5

A normal RPI is 1.0; an RPI of 3.0 or more represents an adequate response of the marrow to anemia. An RPI of <2.0 represents an inadequate response in the presence of anemia.

3. Anemias: The red blood cell indices (MCV, MCHC, MCH) are frequently used to classify anemias (Table 5–2).

Table 5–2. Red blood cell indices in hypochromic and microcytic anemias

	MCV (fl)	MCHC (gm/dL)	MCH (pg)
Normal	83–96	32–36	28–34
Hypochromic	83–100	28–31	23–31
Microcytic	70–82	32–36	22–27
Hypochromic-microcytic	50–79	24–31	11–29

Table 5–3 depicts the laboratory *differentiation of microcytic anemias:*

Table 5–3. Differentiation of microcytic anemias

Abnormality	Ferritin	Serum iron	TIBC	RDW
Chronic disease	N/↑	↓	↓	N
Iron deficiency	↓	↓	↑	↑
Sideroblastic anemia	N/↑	↑	N	N
Thalassemia	N/↑	N/↑	N	N/↑

N = Normal; ↑ = increased; ↓ = decreased; TIBC = total iron binding capacity; RDW = red cell distribution width.

4. **Hemolytic disorders:** Table 5–4 depicts some of the common RBC morphologic abnormalities encountered in patients with *hemolytic disorders.*

5. **Human hemoglobins:** Table 5–5 depicts the normal human hemoglobins at different stages of life.

To convert colorimetric readings into grams of Hb per dL (g/dL) using a standard curve set up with the same equipment and reagents used for the specimen or to calculate specimen concentration (C_u) based on *Beer's law*, the following formula is used:

$$C_u \text{ (g/dL)} = 301 \frac{(A_u \times C_s)}{A_s} \times \frac{1}{1000} = \frac{0.301 \ (A_u \times C_s)}{A_s}$$

where A_u is the absorbance of the unknown; C_s is the concentration of the standard (usually 80 mg/dL); and A_s is the absorbance of the standard run most recently under the same conditions as the patient specimen.

To calculate the fraction of *hemoglobin F as a percentage*, the following formula is used:

$$\text{Hb F (\%)} = \frac{A_{test}}{A_{diluted \ total} \times 5} \times 100$$

where A = absorbance; 5 is the additional dilution factor.

To calculate the *percentage of hemoglobin A₂*:

$$\text{Hb A}_2 \text{ (\% of total)} = \frac{\text{A fraction I}}{\text{A fraction I} + (2.5 \times [\text{A fraction II}])} \times 100\%$$

where A fraction I = absorbance at 415 nm of Hb A_2 eluate after diluting to 10 mL volume; A fraction II = absorbance at 415 nm of eluate (after diluting to 25 mL volume) containing all other hemoglobins after Hb A_2 has been eluted. (Multiplying by a factor of 2.5 corrects for the difference in dilution volumes between fractions I and II).

Table 5-4. Morphologic abnormalities of red blood cells in hemolytic disorders

Abnormality	Hemolytic disorder	
	Congenital	Acquired
Fragmented cells (schistocytes)	Unstable hemoglobins (Heinz body anemias)	Microangiopathic processes Prosthetic heart valves
Permanently sickled cells	Sickle cell anemia	
Spur cells (acanthocytes)	Abetalipoproteinemia	Severe liver disease
Spherocytes	Hereditary spherocytosis	Immune, warm-antibody type
Target cells	Thalassemia Hemoglobinopathies (Hb C)	Liver disease
Agglutinated cells		Immune, cold agglutinin disease

Table 5–5. Normal human hemoglobins at different stages of life

Hemoglobin	Molecular structure	Stage	Proportion (%)	
			Newborns	Adults
Portland	$\zeta_2\gamma_2$	Embryonic	0	0
Gower I	$\zeta_2\epsilon_2$	Embryonic	0	0
Gower II	$\alpha_2\epsilon_2$	Embryonic	0	0
Fetal (F)	$\alpha_2\gamma_2$	Newborn/adult	80	<1
A_1	$\alpha_2\beta_2$	Newborn/adult	20	97
A_2	$\alpha_2\delta_2$	Newborn/adult	<0.5	2.5

6. **Eosinophils:** To calculate the *absolute direct eosinophil count* the following formula can be employed:

$$\text{Eosinophils } (\times\ 10^9/\text{L}) = \frac{\text{Eosinophil count} \times \text{dilution factor}}{\text{Volume counted (mm}^3) \times 10^6}$$

7. **Acquired inhibitors:** Occasionally ICU patients present with acquired inhibitors. The titer of the inhibitors is represented by Bethesda units (BU):

$$1\ \text{BU} = \text{inhibits 1 unit of factor VIII}$$

To calculate the amount of factor VIII required to neutralize the inhibitor and achieve a 50 per cent normal level of circulating factor VIII in a patient who weighs 70 Kg and has a plasma volume of 2800 mL and an inhibitor titer of 10 BU per milliliter, the amount is:

$$2800\ \text{mL} \times 10.5\ \text{BU/mL} = 29{,}400\ \text{BU}$$

8. **Other formulas:** To calculate the *transferrin saturation*, the following formula can be applied:

$$\%\ \text{Transferrin Saturation} = \frac{\text{Serum Iron}}{\text{TIBC}} \times 100$$

For *microscopic cell counting* a Neubauer hemocytometer is needed and the calculation is performed as follows:

$$\text{Cells } (\times\ 10^9/\text{L}) = \frac{\text{Total cells counted} \times \text{Specimen dilution factor}}{\text{mm}^2 \text{ counted} \times 0.1\ \text{mm}} \times 10^6$$

The *plasma volume* is calculated according to the equation:

$$\text{Plasma volume} = \frac{\text{cpm of labeled albumin injected}}{\text{cpm mL plasma at 0 h}}$$

Infectious Diseases

6

Sepsis and its complications constitute one of the leading diagnoses encountered in the critical care setting. The following formulas, facts, and laboratory values are presented as a complement to the practitioner's decisions on diagnosis and management of infectious disease in this setting.

1. **Antibiotic kinetics:** The pharmacokinetics of antibiotics depend on several factors. The *volume of distribution* (V_D) of an antimicrobial is calculated as:

$$V_D = \frac{A}{C_p}$$

where A = total amount of antibiotic in the body; C_p = antibiotic plasma concentration.

Repetitive dosing of antibiotics depends on the principle of *minimal plasma concentrations* (C_{min}):

$$C_{min} = \frac{D}{(V_D)(2^n - 1)}$$

where D = dose; n = dosing interval expressed in half-lives.

The *plasma concentration at steady state* (C_{ss}) of an antimicrobial can be estimated using the following formula:

$$C_{ss} = \frac{\text{Dose per half-life}}{(0.693)(V_D)}$$

2. **Antibiotic adjustments:** Renal dysfunction is common in critically ill patients. In patients receiving aminoglycosides, dosage modification is required according to the *aminoglycoside clearance*:

$$\text{Aminoglycoside clearance} = (C_{cr})\,(0.6) + 10$$

where C_{cr} = creatinine clearance in mL/min.

In order to estimate the *creatinine clearance*, the *Cockcrof and Gault formula* is utilized:

$$C_{cr}(\text{mL/min}) = \frac{(140 - \text{age}) \times \text{weight}}{Cr \times 72}$$

where Cr = serum creatinine in mg/dL. Another modification to this formula is the *Spyker and Guerrant method*:

$$C_{cr}(mL/min) = \frac{(140 - age) \times (1.03 - 0.053 \times Cr)}{Cr}$$

3. **Antibiotic levels:** Some of the clinically employed *antibiotic levels* are depicted in Table 6–1:

Table 6–1.   Levels for selected antibiotics

Antibiotic	Level (μg/mL)	
Amikacin	Peak 20–30	Through <8
Gentamicin	Peak 10–20	Through 5–10
Chloramphenicol	Peak 5–10	Through <2
Tobramycin	Peak 5–10	Through <2
Vancomycin	Peak 30–40	Through 5–10

4. **Other facts:** Some of the *atypical mycobacteria* commonly encountered in the critical care setting are depicted in Table 6–2:

Table 6–2.   Some atypical mycobacteria

Category	Runyon group	Mycobacterial species
Photochromogens	I	*M. kansasii*
		M. marinum
Scotochromogens	II	*M. scrofulaceum*
Nonchromogens	III	*M. avium-intracellulare*
Rapid growers	IV	*M. fortuitum*
		M. chelonae ssp. *chelonae*
		M. chelonae ssp. *abscessus*
		M. ulcerans

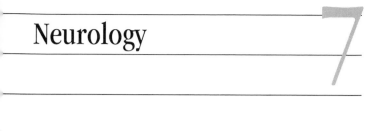

Neurology

Neurologic illness in the intensive care unit may be devastating. The following formulas, facts, and laboratory values may be helpful in the diagnosis and monitoring of neurologic patients.

1. **Cerebrospinal fluid (CSF):** Normal pressures and volumes for *human CSF* are shown in Table 7–1.

Table 7–1. Normal cerebrospinal fluid pressures and volumes

CSF pressure	
Children	3.0–7.5 mm Hg
Adults	3.5–13.5 mm Hg
Volume	
Infants	40–60 mL
Young children	60–100 mL
Older children	80–120 mL
Adult	100–160 mL

The normal *composition of the CSF* is depicted in Table 7–2:

Table 7–2. Normal composition of human cerebrospinal fluid

	CSF concentration (mean)
Specific gravity	1.007
Osmolality (mOsm/Kg H_2O)	289
pH	7.31
PCO_2 (mm Hg)	50.5
Na^+ (mEq/L)	141
K^+ (mEq/L)	2.9
Ca^{++} (mEq/L)	2.5
Mg^{++} (mEq/L)	2.4
Cl^- (mEq/L)	124
Glucose (mg/dL)	61
Protein (mg/dL)	28

Additional normal values for CSF in humans are depicted in Table 7–3:

Table 7–3. Normal cerebrospinal fluid values

CSF parameter	Newborns	Infants, older children, and adults
Leukocyte count	$<32/\mu L$	$<6/\mu L$
Differential white cell count	$<60\%$ polymorphs	<1 polymorph
Proteins	<170 mg/dL	<45 mg/dL
Glucose	>30 mg/dL	>45 mg/dL
CSF: blood/glucose ratio	>0.44	>0.5

In cases of hemorrhage, the white blood cell (WBC) count of the CSF may be dramatically altered. An approximation of the *WBC in blood-contaminated CSF* may be obtained by the formula:

$$\text{Corrected WBC count (CSF)} = \text{WBC (CSF)} - \frac{\text{WBCs (blood)} \times \text{RBC (CSF)}}{\text{RBC (blood)}}$$

When there are many RBCs or WBCs in the CSF, the total protein of the CSF may be "*corrected*" utilizing the following formula:

$$\text{Protein actual} = \text{Protein CSF} - \frac{\text{Protein}_{\text{serum}} \times (1\text{-Hct}) \times \text{RBC}_{\text{CSF}}}{\text{RBC}_{\text{blood}}}$$

The suggested *initial CSF studies* in patients with coma of unknown etiology are depicted in Table 7–4:

Table 7–4. CSF studies in patients with coma of unknown etiology

Tube I
    Cell count with differential
Tube II
    Glucose, protein
Tube III
    Gram's stain, acid-fast bacilli (AFB) stain, routine cultures, India ink and/or cryptococcal antigen, pneumococcal antigen, Venereal Disease Research Laboratories test for syphilis (VDRL)
Tube IV
    Special studies as indicated (e.g., lactic acid, rheumatoid factor)

From Varon J: *Practical Guide to the Care of the Critically Ill Patient.* St. Louis, Mosby–Year Book 205:1994.

The *CSF findings according to etiologic agent* are depicted in Table 7–5:

Table 7–5. Cerebrospinal fluid findings according to etiology

Bacterial	Tuberculous	Viral	Chronic
Glucose <40 mg/dL (blood ratio <0.4)	30–45 mg/dL	20–40 mg/dL	30–40 mg/dL
Protein 100–500 mg/dL	100–500 mg/dL	50–100 mg/dL	100–500 mg/dL
WBC 1000–10,000/cc³	100–400/cm³	10–1000/cm³	100–500/cm³
Gram's stain (+)	AFB smear (+) in up to 40%	Smears are usually negative	Special stains needed India ink capsule (+) 75% AFB (+) 30%
60%–80% (untreated)			
40%–50% (previously treated)			

From Varon J: *Practical Guide to the Care of the Critically Ill Patient.* St. Louis, Mosby–Year Book, 188:1994.

Common CSF abnormalities in patients with *multiple sclerosis* are depicted in Table 7–6:

Table 7–6.   Cerebrospinal fluid abnormalities in multiple sclerosis

	Alb (%)	IgG/TP (%)	IgG/Alb (%)	IgG index (%)	Oligoclonal banding of Ig (%)
Multiple sclerosis	25	67	60–73	70–90	85–95
Normal subjects	3	–	3–6	3	0–7

Alb = albumin; IgG/TP = IgG value/total protein; Ig = immunoglobulin

The abnormalities in IgG production in these patients can be estimated by the *Ig G index:*

$$\text{Ig G index} = \frac{\text{CSF IgG/CSF albumin}}{\text{Serum IgG/serum albumin}} = \text{normal} <0.66$$

2. **Cerebral blood flow:** The cerebral circulation follows the same physiologic principles seen in other circulatory beds, such as the *Ohm's law:*

$$F = \frac{P_i - P_o}{R}$$

where F = flow; P_i = input pressure; P_o = outflow pressure; R = resistance. The term "$P_i - P_o$" is referred to as the cerebral perfusion pressure (CPP).

The *cerebral perfusion pressure* (CPP) can be estimated by the following formula:

$$CPP = MAP - ICP$$

where MAP = mean arterial pressure; ICP = intracranial pressure.

The *pressure-volume index* (PVI) can be calculated as:

$$PVI = \Delta V/[\log P_p/P_o]$$

where P_p = Peak CSF pressure (increase after volume injection and decrease after volume withdrawal).

The *cerebral blood flow* (CQ̇) is normally 50 mL per 100 g per minute and is determined by the *Hagen-Poiseuille equation* of flow through a tube:

$$C\dot{Q} = \frac{(K \times Pr^4)}{(8L \times \eta)}$$

where P = cerebral perfusion pressure (CPP); r = the arterial radius; η = blood viscosity; L = arterial length; K = constant.

To assess the *local cortical cerebral blood flow* (CBF), the following formula can be employed:

$$1CoCBF = \emptyset \frac{(1}{(\Delta V} - \frac{1)}{\Delta Vo)}$$

where ICoCBF = local cortical CBF; Ø = constant value used as a scale factor; ΔVo = maximum temperature difference of zero blood flow; ΔV = actual temperature difference.

To assess flow velocity utilizing transcranial Doppler ultrasound, a resistance index such as the "*pulsatility index*" (PI) can be employed:

$$PI = \frac{\text{Systolic velocity} - \text{diastolic velocity}}{\text{Mean velocity}}$$

3. **Brain metabolism:** *Oxygen availability to neural tissue* (CDO_2) is reflected in the formula:

$$CDO_2 = C\dot{Q} \times Pao_2$$

where $C\dot{Q}$ = cerebral blood flow; Pao_2 = arterial oxygen concentration.

The *cerebral metabolic rate* ($CMRO_2$) can be calculated as:

$$CMRO_2 = CBF \times A V\dot{D}O_2$$

where CBF = cerebral blood flow; $A V\dot{D}O_2$ = arteriovenous oxygen content difference.

The *oxygen extraction ratio* (OER) can be utilized to assess the brain metabolism:

$$OER = SaO_2 - Sj\overline{v}O_2/SaO_2$$

where SaO_2 = arterial oxygen saturation; $Sj\overline{v}O_2$ = jugular venous oxygen saturation.

$$OER \times CaO_2 = CMRO_2/CBF$$

where

$$CaO_2 = (Hb \times 1.39 \times SaO_2) + [0.003 \times Po_2 \text{ (mm Hg)}]$$

$$CMRO_2 = CBF \times (CaO_2 - Cj\overline{v}O_2)$$

The *arterial-jugular venous oxygen content difference* ($Aj\overline{v}\dot{D}O_2$) is calculated as:

$$Aj\overline{v}\dot{D}O_2 = CMRO_2/CBF$$

4. Miscellaneous: The *Glasgow coma scale* (GCS) is commonly used in critically ill patients and is depicted in Table 7–7:

Table 7–7.   Glasgow coma scale

	Score
Eye Opening	
Spontaneous	4
To verbal command	3
To pain	2
None	1
Best Motor Response	
Obeys verbal command	6
Localizes painful stimuli	5
Flexion withdrawal from painful stimuli	4
Decorticate (flexion) response to painful stimuli	3
Decerebrate (extension) response to painful stimuli	2
None	1
Best Verbal Response	
Oriented conversation	5
Disoriented conversation	4
Inappropriate words	3
Incomprehensible sounds	2
None	1

TOTAL SCORE: 3–15

From Teasdale G, Jennett B: Assessment of coma and impaired consciousness: a practical scale. *Lancet* 1974; 2:81–3.

The *apnea test* can be performed following the instructions shown in Table 7–8:

Table 7–8.   The Apnea test

1. Oxygenate with 100% FiO_2 for 5–10 min before the test
2. Keep O_2 at 4–8 L/min delivered through a canula in the endotracheal tube while the patient is disconnected from the ventilator.* (If hypotension and/or dysrhythmias develop, immediately reconnect to the ventilator. Consider other confirmatory tests)
3. Observe for spontaneous respirations
4. After 10 min, obtain arterial blood gases (ABG). Patient is apneic if $Pco_2 \geq 60$ torr and there are no respiratory movements

*In patients with chronic obstructive pulmonary disease (COPD), the PaO_2 must be <50 torr at the end of the apnea test.

(From Varon J: *Practical Guide to the Care of the Critically Ill Patient.* St. Louis, Mosby–Year Book, 204:1994.)

Nutrition

Adequate nutrition is of paramount importance to optimal survival from critical illness. Many patients in intensive care units cannot or will not take adequate nutrition orally; thus, supplementation of nutrients via alternative enteral or parenteral routes may be important. The following facts and formulas represent the information necessary for assessment and administration of nutritional support.

1. **Nutritional assessment:** The *total daily energy* (TDE) requirements for a patient can be calculated using the following formula:

$$\text{TDE for men (kcal/day)} = (66.47 + 13.75W + 5.0H - 6.76A)$$
$$\times \text{(Activity factor)} \times \text{(Injury factor)}$$

$$\text{TDE for women (kcal/day)} = (655.10 + 9.56W + 1.85H - 4.68A)$$
$$\times \text{(Activity factor)} \times \text{(Injury factor)}$$

where W = weight (Kg), H = height (cm), A = age (years); the activity factor is derived from Table 8–1.

Table 8–1. Activity factor

Confined to bed	1.2
Out of bed	1.3

The *injury factors* can be estimated based on Table 8–2.

The *metabolic rate* (MR) can be calculated in patients with a pulmonary artery catheter as:

$$\text{MR (kcal/hr)} = \dot{V}O_2 \text{ (mL/min)} \times 60 \text{ min/hr}$$
$$\times 1 \text{ L/1,000 mL} \times 4.83 \text{ kcal/L}$$

where $\dot{V}O_2$ (mL/min) = Cardiac output (L/min) × [arterial oxygen content (CaO_2, mL/L) − mixed venous oxygen content (CmO_2, mL/L)]

Table 8–2.   Injury factors

Surgery	
Minor	1.0–1.1
Major	1.1–1.2
Infection	
Mild	1.0–1.2
Moderate	1.2–1.4
Severe	1.4–1.8
Trauma	
Skeletal	1.2–1.35
Head injury with steroid therapy	1.6
Blunt	1.15–1.35
Burns (body surface area)	
Up to 20%	1.0–1.5
20% to 40%	1.5–1.85
Over 40%	1.85–1.95

The *prognostic nutritional index* (PNI) allows for nutritional assessment of the critically ill patient and is calculated as:

$$\text{PNI} (\% \text{ risk}) = 158\% - 16.6 \text{ (alb)} - 0.78 \text{ (TSF)} - 0.2 \text{ (tfn)} - 5.8 \text{ (DSH)}$$

where alb = serum albumin (gm/dL); TSF = triceps skin fold (mm); tfn = serum transferrin (mg/dL); DSH = delayed skin hypersensitivity (1 = anergy, 2 = reactive)

The *probability of survival* (POS) based on the nutritional status of a critically ill patient can be calculated as:

$$\text{POS} = 0.91 \text{ (alb)} - 1.0 \text{ (DSH)} - 1.44 \text{ (SEP)} + 0.98 \text{ (DIA)} - 1.09$$

where alb = serum albumin (gm/dL); DSH = delayed skin hypersensitivity (1 = anergy, 2 = reactive); SEP = sepsis (1 = no sepsis, 2 = sepsis); DIA = diagnosis of cancer (1 = no cancer, 2 = cancer)

Another way to calculate the nutritional deficit is by utilizing the *index of undernutrition* (IOU) (Table 8–3).

Table 8–3.   Index of undernutrition

	Points				
Assay	0	5	10	15	20
Albumin (g/dL)	>3.5	3.1–3.5	2.6–3.0	2.0–2.5	<2.0
Fat area (%)	>70	56–70	46–55	30–45	<30
Muscle area (%)	>80	76–80	61–75	40–60	<40
Transferrin (g/L)	>2.0	1.76–2.0	1.41–1.75	1.0–1.4	<40
Weight lost (%)	0	0–10	11–14	15–20	>20

The calculation of *daily protein requirements* (PR) can be done utilizing the following formula:

PR (gms) = (Patient weight) in Kg × (PR for illness in g/Kg)

In order to determine the *nonprotein caloric requirements* (NCR):

NCR = (Total required calories) − (Required protein calories)

The *nitrogen balance* (NB) reflects the status of the net protein use:

NB = (Dietary protein × 0.16) − (UUN + 2 g stool + 2 g skin)

where UUN = urine urea nitrogen.

In patients with renal failure, the increased blood urea pool and extrarenal urea losses must be accounted for:

NB = Nitrogen in − (UUN + 2 g stool + 2 g skin + BUN change)

In addition to the above formulas, the *catabolic index* (CI) can be derived from the same variables:

CI = UUN − [(0.5 × Dietary protein × 0.16) + 3 g]

No nutritional stress results in a CI ≤ 0, in moderate nutritional stress CI <5, and in severe nutritional stress >5.

Another index of the loss of lean tissue in malnourished patients is the *creatinine height index* (CHI), which can be calculated as:

CHI = Measured creatinine/expected creatinine

The *body mass index* (BMI) normalizes for height and allows comparisons among diverse populations:

BMI = Body weight (Kg)/(height)^2 (m)

The *Harris-Benedict equation* (HBE) is frequently utilized in assessment of the basal energy expenditure (BEE):

HBE BEE = 66 + (13.7 × (5 × H) − 6.8 × A) males
= 665 + (9.6 × W) + (1.7 × H) − (4.7 × A) females

where W = weight (Kg); H = height (cm); A = age (years).

2. **Fuel composition:** The body uses different sources of fuel. Table 8–4 depicts some of them.

3. **Other formulas:** The *body surface area* (BSA) of a patient can be calculated as:

$$BSA \ (m^2) = \frac{(Weight \ in \ Kg)^{0.425} \times (height \ in \ cm)^{0.725} \times 71.84}{10,000}$$

The *ideal body weight* (IBW) for height in males and females can be estimated based on Table 8–5.

Table 8–4. Normal fuel composition of the human body

Fuel	Amount (Kg)	Calories (kcal)
Circulating fuels		
Glucose	0.020	80
Free fatty acids (plasma)	0.0003	3
Triglycerides (plasma)	0.003	30
Total		113
Tissue		
Fat (adipose triglycerides)	15	141,000
Protein (muscle)	6	24,000
Glycogen (muscle)	0.150	600
Glycogen (liver)	0.075	300
Total		165,900

Table 8–5. Ideal body weight in males and females

Height in cm	Males (*Weight in Kg*)	Females (*Weight in Kg*)
145	51.8	47.5
150	54.5	50.4
155	57.2	53.1
160	60.5	56.2
165	63.5	59.5
175	70.1	66.3
180	74.2	
185	78.1	

The *percentage of ideal body weight* (%IBW) is calculated as:

$$\%IBW = \frac{100 \times (height\ in\ cm)}{IBW}$$

Obstetrics and Gynecology

In most instances female ICU patients are managed the same way as male patients. The issues of pregnancy and medical conditions unique to women, of course, create exceptions. The following tables and formulas should be useful to the practitioner caring for pregnant patients.

1. **Hemodynamics:** The hemodynamic changes that occur in pregnancy are depicted in Tables 9–1 and 9–2:

Table 9–1. Hemodynamic changes of pregnancy

Parameter	Change
Cardiac output	Increases 30%–40%
Heart rate	Increase 10–15 BPM
Stroke volume	Increases
Blood volume	Increases 30%–40%
Systemic blood pressure	Decreases
Pulse pressure	Increases
Systemic resistance	Decreases
Pulmonary artery pressure	No change
Pulmonary resistance	Decreases
Myocardial function	Improves

From Varon J: *Practical Guide to the Care of the Critically Ill Patient.* St. Louis, Mosby–Year Book, 253:1994.

Table 9–2. Hemodynamic effects of labor and delivery

Parameter	Effect
Cardiac output	Increases with contractions
Blood volume	Increases
Heart rate	Variable
Peripheral resistance	No change
Systemic artery pressure	Increases

From Varon J: *Practical Guide to the Care of the Critically Ill Patient.* St. Louis, Mosby–Year Book, 253:1994.

The hemodynamic responses expected in response to position changes in the third trimester of pregnancy are depicted in Table 9–3:

Table 9–3. Hemodynamic alterations in response to position change late in third trimester of pregnancy

Hemodynamic parameter	Position			
	Left lateral	Supine	Sitting	Standing
MAP (mm Hg)	90 ± 6	90 ± 8	90 ± 8	91 ± 14
Cardiac output (L/min)	6.6 ± 1.4	6.0 ± 1.4*	6.2 ± 2.05	4 ± 2.0*
Pulse (bpm)	82 ± 10	84 ± 10	91 ± 11	107 ± 17*
Systemic vascular resistance (dyne/cm/sec^{-5})	1210 ± 266	1437 ± 338	1217 ± 254	1319 ± 394
Pulmonary vascular resistance (dyne/cm/sec^{-5})	76 ± 16	101 ± 45	102 ± 35	117 ± 35*
Pulmonary capillary wedge pressure (mm Hg)	8 ± 2	6 ± 3	4 ± 4	4 ± 2
Central venous pressure (mm Hg)	4 ± 3	3 ± 2	1 ± 1	1 ± 2
Left ventricular stroke word index (g/m/m²/beat)	43 ± 9	40 ± 9	44 ± 5	34 ± 7*

*Pulse <0.05, compared with left lateral position.
Modified from Clark SL, Cotton DB, Pivarnik JM, et al: Position change and central hemodynamic profile during normal third-trimester pregnancy and postpartum. *Am J Obstet Gynecol* 1991; 164:883–7.

Uterine oxygen consumption can be calculated by the following formula:

$$O_2 \text{ Uptake by Gravid Uterus} = (A - V) \times F$$

where A = maternal arterial blood oxygen content, V = uterine venous blood oxygen content, F = uterine blood flow.

The *oxygen saturation of the uterine venous blood flow* (Sv) is another important parameter to follow and is calculated as:

$$Sv = \frac{SaO_2 - \dot{V}O_2}{F \times (O_2\ Cap)}$$

where SaO_2 = maternal oxygen saturation, $\dot{V}O_2$ = oxygen consumption rate, F = uterine blood flow, O_2 Cap = oxygen capacity of maternal blood.

2. **Pulmonary:** The changes in pulmonary function expected during pregnancy are depicted in Table 9–4:

Table 9–4. Lung volumes and capacities in pregnancy

	Definition	Change in pregnancy
Respiratory rate (RR)	Number of breaths per min (bpm)	Unchanged
Vital capacity (VC)	Maximum amount of air that can be forcibly expired after maximum inspiration (IC + ERV)	Unchanged
Inspiratory capacity (IC)	Maximum amount of air that can be inspired from resting expiratory level (TV + IRV)	Increased 5%
Tidal volume (VT)	Amount of air inspired and expired with normal breath	Increased 30%–40%
Inspiratory reserve volume (IRV)	Maximum amount of air that can be inspired at end of normal inspiration	Unchanged
Functional residual capacity (FRC)	Amount of air in lungs at resting expiratory level (ERV + RV)	Decreased 20%
Expiratory reserve volume (ERV)	Maximum amount of air that can be expired from resting expiratory level	Decreased 20%
Residual volume (RV)	Amount of air in lungs after maximum expiration	Decreased 20%
Total lung capacity (TLC)	Total amount of air in lungs at maximal inspiration (VC + RV)	Decreased 5%

From Cruikshank DP, Hays PM: *Maternal physiology in pregnancy.* In Gabbe SG, Niebyl JR, Simpson JL, editors: *Obstetrics: normal and problem pregnancies,* ed 2, New York, 1991, Churchill Livingstone.

3. **Other formulas:** If the last menstrual period (LMP) is known, the probable delivery date (DD) can be approximated utilizing *Naegele's rule*:

$$DD = \text{First day of LMP} + 7 \text{ days} - 3 \text{ months}$$

The approximate *weight gain* (WG) by a pregnant woman can be calculated after the second trimester as:

$$WG = 225 \text{ gm} \times \text{weeks of gestation}$$

Occasionally there is a need for *intraperitoneal fetal transfusion* in a gravid patient. The following formula is used to calculate the volume of red blood cells (RBC) to be injected into the fetal peritoneal cavity (IPT volume):

$$IPT \text{ volume} = (\text{weeks' gestation} - 20) \times 10 \text{ mL}.$$

To determine the concentration of donor hemoglobin present in the fetus at any time following an intrauterine transfusion, *Bowman's formula* is applied:

$$Hb \text{ concentration (gm/dL)} = \frac{0.55 \times a}{85 \times b} \times \frac{120 - c}{120}$$

where 0.55 = fraction of transfused RBC in the fetal circulation, a = amount of donor RBC transfused (grams), b = fetal weight (Kg), c = interval (days) from the time of transfusion to the time of calculation, 85 = estimation of blood volume (mL/Kg) in the fetus, 120 = life span of donor RBC.

The *placental transfer of drugs* can be calculated as:

$$Q/t = \frac{KA \, (C_m - C_f)}{D}$$

Q/t = rate of diffusion, K = diffusion constant, A = surface area available for exchange, C_m = concentration of free drug in maternal blood, C_f = concentration of free drug in fetal blood, D = thickness of diffusion barrier.

Oncology

10

Cancer patients comprise a large portion of those needing critical care services. Some may require critical care on a short-term basis for the complications of their underlying malignant disease; others need aggressive antineoplastic therapy. The following formulas and facts will aid the clinician in the diagnosis and management of these patients.

1. **Basic oncology formulas:** Although not critically useful, these formulas allow a better understanding of the oncogenesis process, its complications, and the response to therapy.

   The rapidly proliferating component of human tumors is known as the *growth factor* (GF) and is calculated as:

$$GF = \frac{\text{Observed fraction of cells in S}}{\text{Expected fraction of cells in S}}$$

   where S = part of cell cycle where DNA synthesis occurs predominantly.

   The fraction of cells in "S" phase can be assessed by titrated thymidine labeling and autoradiography. The fraction of labeled cells is known as the *thymidine labeling index* (TLI):

$$TLI = \frac{\text{Number of labeled cells}}{\text{Total number of cells}}$$

2. **Nutrition in cancer:** Also refer to Chapter 8 (Nutrition). Cancer patients are frequently malnourished and require close nutritional monitoring. To assess the amount of weight loss (*percent weight change*) that these patients have the following formula is utilized:

$$\text{Percent weight change} = \frac{(\text{Usual weight} - \text{Actual weight})}{(\text{Usual weight})} \times 100$$

The evaluation of weight change based on the percent weight change formula is depicted in Table 10–1:

Table 10–1. Evaluation of weight change based on the percent weight change formula

	Significant weight loss (%)	Severe weight loss (%)
7 days	1–2	>2
1 month	5	>5
3 months	7.5	>7.5
6 months	10	>10

A useful formula in the nutritional assessment of these patients relates to the *nitrogen balance:*

$$\text{Nitrogen balance} = \frac{\text{Protein intake (g)}}{6.25} - (24\text{-h urine urea nitrogen} + 4 \text{ g})$$

The *catabolic index* (CI) aids in the identification of the amount of "nutritional stress" that these patients have:

CI = 24h urine nitrogen excretion − [½ dietary nitrogen (g) intake + 3]

The interpretation of the Catabolic index is depicted in Table 10–2:

Table 10–2. Interpretation of the catabolic index

Catabolic index	Interpretation
0	No significant stress
1–5	Mild stress
>5	Moderate to severe stress

The *arm muscle circumference* (AMC) is another sensitive measure of protein nutritional status in cancer patients:

AMC = Arm circumference − (TSF)

where TSF = triceps skinfold measurement.

3. Other facts: The cerebrospinal fluid (CSF) findings in patients with *carcinomatous meningitis* are depicted in Table 10–3:

Table 10–3.   CSF findings in patients with carcinomatous meningitis

Parameter	Percent of abnormal patients	Range
Opening pressure	50	60–450
WBC count	52	0–1800
Glucose	30–38	0–244
Protein	30–81	24–2485
Cytology	41–70	24–2485

Pericardial tamponade represents one of the complications that can occur in cancer patients. Its hemodynamic interpretation is depicted in Table 10–4.

The *body surface area* (BSA) of a patient can be calculated as:

$$\text{BSA (m}^2) = \frac{(\text{Weight in Kg})^{0.425} \times (\text{height in cm})^{0.725} \times 71.84}{10,000}$$

Table 10-4. Hemodynamic parameters of pericardial tamponade and pericardial constriction

	Pericardial tamponade	Pericardial constriction
Right atrial pressure	≥15 mm Hg	≥15 mm Hg usually with prominent "y" trough
Left atrial pressure	Equals right atrial pressure	Equals right atrial pressure
Right ventricular pressure	No diastolic dip	Consistent early
Right ventricular diastolic pressure	≤1/3 systolic blood pressure	≥1/3 systolic right ventricular pressure
Pulmonary artery pressure	Systolic pulmonary artery pressure often ≤40 mm Hg	Systolic pulmonary artery pressure <40 mm Hg
Cardiac output	Decreased	Usually normal with normal arteriovenous difference
Respiratory variation in pressure	Usually present	Absent
Diastolic pressures	Equal	Equal

Pediatrics

In no other area of critical care are formulas as important as in pediatrics. The large variation in patient size requires that simple rules of thumb be available to the critical care practitioner.

1. **Airways:** Selecting the proper *size* (internal diameter [ID]) endotracheal tube (ETT) in children is important. The most commonly utilized formula is that of *Cole*:

$$\text{Tube size (mm ID)} = \frac{\text{Age (yr)}}{4} + 4$$

or

$$\text{Tube size (mm ID)} = \frac{16 + \text{Age (yr)}}{4}$$

The estimation of the *ETT in newborns* can be accomplished by the following formula:

$$\text{Tube size (mm ID)} = \frac{\text{Postconceptual age in weeks}}{10}$$

The proper *distance for insertion* of endotracheal tubes in children older than 2 years can be approximated by the following formulas:

$$\text{Distance (cm)} = \frac{\text{Age (yr)}}{2} + 12$$

or

$$\text{Depth of insertion} = \text{ETT ID} \times 3$$

2. **Hemodynamics:** Normal blood pressure values vary according to age. The *median systolic blood pressure* (SBP) for children older than 1 year is approximated by the following formula:

$$\text{SBP} = 90 \text{ mm Hg} + (2 \times \text{age in years})$$

The *lower limit* of the SBP (SBP$_{LL}$) can be estimated as:

$$SBP_{LL} = 70 \text{ mm Hg} + (2 \times \text{age in years})$$

The *diastolic blood pressure* (DBP) calculation is:

$$DBP = 2/3 \text{ systolic blood pressure}$$

The *normal heart rate* (HR) varies according to age. Table 11–1 depicts normal heart rate at different age groups:

Table 11–1.   Heart rate at different age intervals

Age	Heart rate/min
0–1 month	100–180 (150)
2–3 months	110–180 (120)
4–12 months	100–180 (150)
1–3 years	100–180 (130)
4–5 years	60–150 (100)
6–8 years	60–130 (100)
9–11 years	50–110 (80)
12–16 years	50–100 (75)
> 16 years	50–90 (70)

3. **Intravenous cannulation:** The equipment necessary varies according to the age and weight of the pediatric critical care patient. Below is a comparison table of different gauges for *over-the-needle catheters* for pediatric patients (Table 11–2).

Table 11–2.   Catheter gauge for over-the-needle cannulation in pediatric critically ill patients

Age (years)	Weight (Kg)	Gauge
<1	<10	20, 22, 24
1–12	10–40	16, 18, 20
>12	>40	14, 16, 18

For *umbilical vein catheterization* it is important to have a precise catheter length in order to place this catheter in the inferior vena cava. The following formula can be used for this estimation:

$$UV \text{ catheter length (cm)} = [0.5 \times UA \text{ catheter length (cm)}] + 1$$

4. **Nutrition:** Estimating the *body weight* in children can be done utilizing the following formula:

$$\text{Estimated body weight (Kg)} = (\text{age in years} \times 2) + 8$$

The *energy needs* (basal metabolic rate or BMR) for a pediatric patient can be calculated using the following formulas:

$$\text{BMR males} = 66 + (13.7 \times W) + (5.0 \times H) - (6.8 \times A)$$
$$\text{BMR females} = 665 + (9.6 \times W) + (1.7 \times H) - (4.7 \times A)$$

where W = weight in kilograms, H = height in centimeters, A = age in years.
To evaluate the *nutritional stress* of the pediatric patient in the intensive care unit, the catabolic index (CI) can be used:

$$CI = UUN - (0.5 \times N_{in} + 3)$$

where UUN = 24 hour urine urea nitrogen in grams, N_{in} = 24 hour nitrogen intake in grams.
For additional formulas, please refer to Chapter 8.

5. **Water requirements:** *Water requirements* for children vary according to the age and weight of the child (Table 11–3).

Table 11–3. Maintenance fluid requirements of children

Weight	Maintenance fluids
Less than 10 Kg	100 mL/Kg/24 h
11 to 20 Kg	1000 mL + 50 mL/Kg/24 h for each Kg over 10 Kg
More than 20 Kg	1500 mL + 20 mL/Kg/24 h for each Kg over 20 Kg

6. **Cation requirements:** Daily major *cation requirements* in the youngsters can be summarized as follows:

$$Na^+ = 3 \text{ mEq/Kg/24 h (maximum 80 mEq/24 h)}$$
$$K^+ = 2 \text{ mEq/Kg/24 h (maximum 40 mEq/24 h)}$$

7. **Urinary water losses:** *Urinary losses* (UL) reflect the solute load, excretion and urine concentration:

$$UL = 60 \text{ mL/Kg/24 h}$$

8. **Fecal water losses:** In general, *fecal losses* (FL) are small in young children and insignificant in older children:

$$FL = 10 \text{ mL/Kg/24 h}$$

9. **Insensible water losses:** *Insensible losses* (IL) mostly occur through skin and respiratory tract:

$$IL = 30 \text{ mL/Kg/24 h}$$

Fever increases IL by 7 mL/Kg/24 h for each degree rise in temperature above $37.2°$ C ($99°$ F).

10. **Hematologic formulas:** In order to estimate the *required packed cell volume*, use the formula:

$$\text{Vol of cells (ml)} = \frac{\text{Estimated blood volume (ml)} \times \text{Desired Hct change}}{\text{Hct of PRBC}}$$

In patients with severe anemia, *rapid correction of the hemoglobin* can be achieved utilizing the formula:

$$\text{Volume (ml)} = \frac{\text{Blood volume (ml)} \times \text{Desired Hb rise}}{22 \text{ g/dL} - \text{HbR}}$$

where

$$\text{HbR} = \frac{\text{Initial Hb} - \text{Desired Hb}}{2}$$

In pediatric patients undergoing *exchange transfusion*, the following formula can be applied:

$$V = \frac{(\text{Hct}_i - \text{Hct}_f) \times \text{Body weight (Kg)} \times 70 \text{ mL/Kg}}{\text{Hct}_i}$$

where V = volume to be exchanged, Hct_i = initial hematocrit, Hct_f = final hematocrit.

11. **Other formulas:** Occasionally it is necessary to calculate the *stool osmotic gap* (SOG) to determine the type of diarrhea (i.e., secretory, malabsorption, etc.). The stool osmotic gap can be calculated with the formula:

$$\text{SOG} = 290 - 2 \times ([Na^+] \times [K^+])$$

The formula used to calculate the rate of *glucose infusion in neonates* is:

$$\text{Glucose infusion (mg/Kg/min glucose)} = \frac{(\% \text{ glucose in solution} \times 10) \times \text{rate of infusion})}{60 \times \text{weight (Kg)}}$$

12. **Selected pediatric laboratory values:** Blood = (B), Serum = (S), Plasma = (P), Urine = (U), Red blood cells = (RBC)

Acid-Base Measurements (B)
pH: 7.38–7.42 from 14 minutes of age and older.
Pao_2: 65–76 mm Hg (8.66–10.13 kPa).
$Paco_2$: 36–38 mm Hg (4.8–5.07 kPa).
Base excess: -2 to $+2$ mEq/L, except in newborns

Acid Phosphatase (S,P)

Values using p-nitrophenyl phosphate buffered with citrate.
Newborns: 7.4–19.4 IU/L at 37°C
2–13 years: 6.4–15.2 IU/L at 37°C
Adult males: 0.5–11 IU/L at 37°C
Adult females: 0.2–9.5 IU/L at 37°C

Alanine Aminotransferase (ALAT, ALT, SGPT) (S)

Newborns (1–3 days): 1–25 UI/L at 37°C
Adult males: 7–46 IU/L at 37°C
Adult females: 4–35 IU/L at 37°C

Aldolase (S)

Newborns: 17.5–47.8 UI/L at 37°C
Children: 8.8–23.9 IU/L at 37°C
Adults: 4.4–12 IU/L at 37°C

Ammonia (P)

Newborns: 90–150 μg/dL (53–88 μmol/L); higher in premature and
jaundiced infants; thereafter 0–60 μg/dL (0–35 μmol/L) when blood is
drawn with proper precautions.

Amylase

Values using maltotetrose substrate (kinetic)
Neonates: Undetectable
2–12 months: Levels increase slowly to adult levels
Adults: 28–108 IU/L at 37°C

Aspartate Aminotransferase (ASAT, AST, SGOT) (S)

Newborns (1–3 days): 16–74 IU/L at 37°C
Adult males: 8–46 IU/L at 37°C
Adult females: 7–34 IU/L at 37°C

Bicarbonate, Actual (P)

Calculated from pH and $Paco_2$
Newborns: 17.2–23.6 mmol/L
2 months–2 years: 19–24 mmol/L
Children: 18–25 mmol/L
Adult males: 20.1–28.9 mmol/L
Adult females: 18.4–28.8 mmol/L

Bilirubin (S)

Levels after 1 month are as follows:
Conjugated: 0–0.3 mg/dL (0–5 μmol/L)
Unconjugated: 0.1–0.7 mg/dL (2–12 μmol/L)

Bleeding Time (Simplate)

2–9 minutes

Blood Volume
Premature infants: 98 mL/Kg
At 1 year: 86 mL/Kg (range, 69–112 mL/Kg)
Older children: 70 mL/Kg (range, 51–86 mL/Kg)

Calcium (S)
Premature infants (first week) 3.5–4.5 mEq/L (1.7–2.3 mmol/L)
Full-term infants (first week): 4–5 mEq/L (2–2.5 mmol/L)
Thereafter: 4.4–5.3 mEq/L (2.2–2.7 mmol/L)

Carbon Dioxide, Total (S,P)
Umbilical cord blood: 15–20.2 mmol/L
Children: 18–27 mmol/L
Adults: 24–35 mmol/L

Carboxyhemoglobin (B)
5% of total hemoglobin

Chloride (S,P)
Premature infants: 95–110 mmol/L
Full-term infants: 96–116 mmol/L
Children: 98–105 mmol/L
Adults: 98–108 mmol/L

Cholesterol, Total (S,P) (Table 11–4)
Values in mg/dL (mmol/L)

Table 11–4. Cholesterol values in childhood

Age group (years)	Value for males	Values for females
6–7	115–197 (2.97–5.09)	126–199 (3.25–5.14)
8–9	112–199 (2.89–5.14)	124–208 (3.20–5.37)
10–11	108–220 (2.79–5.68)	115–208 (2.97–5.37)
12–13	117–202 (3.02–5.21)	114–207 (2.94–5.34)
14–15	103–207 (2.66–5.34)	102–208 (2.63–5.37)
16–17	107–198 (2.76–5.11)	106–213 (2.73–5.50)

Cortisol (S,P)
Morning (8:00 AM): 5–25 μg/dL (0.14–0.68 μmol/L)
Evening: 5–15 μg/dL (0.14–0.41 μmol/L)

Creatine Kinase (S,P)
Newborns (1–3 days): 40–474 IU/L at 37°C
Adult males: 30–210 IU/L at 37°C
Adult females: 20–128 IU/L at 37°C

Creatinine (S,P) (Table 11–5)
Values in mg/dL (μmol/L)

Table 11–5. Normal creatinine values in childhood

Age group	Values for males	Values for females
Newborns (1–3 days)*	0.2–1.0 (17.7–88.4)	0.2–1.0 (17.7–88.4)
1 year	0.2–0.6 (17.7–53.0)	0.2–0.5 (17.7–44.2)
2–3 years	0.2–0.7 (17.7–61.9)	0.3–0.6 (26.5–53.0)
4–7 years	0.2–0.8 (17.7–70.7)	0.2–0.7 (17.7–61.9)
8–10 years	0.3–0.9 (26.5–79.6)	0.3–0.8 (26.5–70.7)
11–12 years	0.3–1.0 (26.5–88.4)	0.3–0.9 (26.5–79.6)
13–17 years	0.3–1.2 (26.5–106.1)	0.3–1.1 (26.5–97.2)

*Values may be higher in premature newborns.

Creatinine Clearance
Newborns (1–6 days): 5–50 mL/min/1.73 m^2 (mean, 18 mL/min/1.73 m^2).
Newborns (>6 days): 15–90 mL/min/1.73 m^2 (mean 36 mL/min/1.73 m^2)
Adult males: 85–125 mL/min/1.73 m^2
Adult females: 75–115 mL/min/1.73 m^2

Fibrinogen (P)
200–500 mg/dL (5.9–14.7 μmol/L)

Glomerular Filtration Rate
Newborns: About 50% of values for older children and adults
Older children and adults: 75–165 mL/min/1.73 m^2 (levels reached by about 6 months)

Haptoglobin (S)
50–150 mg/dL has hemoglobin-binding capacity.

Hematocrit (B)
At birth: 44%–64%
14–90 days: 35%–49%
6 months–1 year: 30%–40%
4–10 years: 31%–43%

Lactate (B)
Venous blood: 5–18 mg/dL (0.5–2 mmol/L)
Arterial blood: 3–7 mg/dL (0.3–0.8 mmol/L)

Lactate Dehydrogenase (LDH) (S,P)
Newborns (1–3 days): 40–348 IU/L at 37°C
1 month–5 years: 150–360 IU/L at 37°C
5–8 years: 150–300 IU/L at 37°C
8–12 years: 130–300 IU/L at 37°C

12–14 years: 130–280 IU/L at 37°C
14–16 years: 130–230 IU/L at 37°C
Adult males: 70–178 IU/L at 37°C
Adult females: 42–166 IU/L at 37°C

Lactate Dehydrogenase Isoenzymes (S)
LDH_1 (heart): 24%–34%
LDH_2 (heart, red blood cells): 35%–45%
LDH_3 (muscle): 15%–25%
LDH_4 (liver [trace], muscle) 4%–10%
LDH_5 (liver, muscle): 1%–9%

Lead (B)
<10 μg/dL (<0.48 μmol/L)

Lipase (S,P)
20–136 IU/L based on 4-h incubation

Magnesium (S,P)
Newborn: 1.5–2.3 mEq/L (0.75–1.15 mmol/L)
Adults: 1.4–2 mEq/L (0.7–1 mmol/L)

Magnesium (RBC)
3.92–5.28 mEq/L (1.96–2.64 mmol/L)

Manganese (S)
Newborns: 2.4–9.6 μg/dL (0.44–1.75 μmol/L)
Adults: 1.4–2 μg/dL (0.15–0.38 μmol/L)

Methemoglobin (B)
0–0.3 g/dL (0–186 μmol/L)

Osmolality (S,P)
270–290 mOsm/Kg

Oxygen Capacity (B)
1.34 mL/g of hemoglobin

Oxygen Saturation [Venous] (B)
Newborns: 30%–80% (0.3–0.8 mol/mol of venous blood)
Thereafter: 65%–85% (0.65–0.85 mol/mol of venous blood)

Partial Thromboplastin Time (P)
Children: 42–54 seconds

Phosphorus, Inorganic (S,P)
Premature infants:
   At birth: 5.6–8 mg/dL (1.81–2.58 mmol/L)
   6–10 days: 6.1–11.7 mg/dL (1.97–3.78 mmol/L)
   20–25 days: 6.6–9.4 mg/dL (2.13–3.04 mmol/L)
Full-term infants:
   At birth: 5–7.8 mg/dL (1.61–2.52 mmol/L)
   3 days: 5.8–9 mg/dL (1.87–2.91 mmol/L)
   6–12 days: 4.9–8.9 mg/dL (1.58–2.87 mmol/L)

Children:
   1 year: 3.8–6.2 mg/dL (1.23–2 mmol/L)
   10 years: 3.6–5.6 mg/dL (1.16–1.81 mmol/L)

Potassium (S,P)
Premature infants: 4.5–7.2 mmol/L
Full-term infants: 3.7–5.2 mmol/L
Children: 3.5–5.8 mmol/L
Adults: 3.5–5.5 mmol/L

Potassium (RBC)
Children: 87.2–97.6 mmol/L

Prothrombin Time (P)
Children: 11–15 seconds

Sedimentation Rate (B)
<2 years: 1–5 mm/h
>2 years: 1–8 mm/h

Sodium (S,P)
Children and adults: 135–148 mmol/L

Thrombin Time (P)
Children: 12–16 sec

Triglyceride (S,P) (Table 11–6)
Fasting (>12 h) values in mg/mL (mmol/L):

Table 11–6.   Fasting triglyceride values in childhood

Age group (years)	Values for males	Values for females
6–7	32–79 (0.36–0.89)	24–128 (0.27–1.44)
8–9	28–105 (0.31–1.18)	34–115 (0.38–1.29)
10–11	30–115 (0.33–1.29)	39–131 (0.44–1.48)
12–13	33–112 (0.37–1.26)	36–125 (0.40–1.41)
14–15	35–136 (0.39–1.53)	36–122 (0.40–1.37)
16–17	38–167 (0.42–1.88)	34–136 (0.38–1.53)

Urea Nitrogen (S,P)
1–2 years: 5–15 mg/dL (1.8–5.4 mmol/L)
Thereafter: 10–20 mg/dL (3.5–7.1 mmol/L)

Uric Acid (S,P)
Males:
   0–14 years: 2–7 mg/dL (119–416 μmol/L)
   >14 years: 3–8 mg/dL (178–476 μmol/L)
Females:
   0–14 years: 2–7 mg/dL (119–416 μmol/L)
   >14 years: 2–7 mg/dL (119–416 μmol/L)

Volume (B)
Premature infants: 98 mL/Kg (mean)
Full-term infants: 75–100 mL/Kg
1 year: 69–112 mL/Kg (mean, 86 mL/Kg)
Older children: 51–86 mL/Kg (mean, 70 mL/Kg)

Volume (P)
Full-term neonates: 39–77 mL/Kg
Infants: 40–50 mL/Kg
Older children: 30–54 mL/Kg

Water (B,S,RBC)
Whole blood: 79–81 g/dL
Serum: 91–92 g/dL

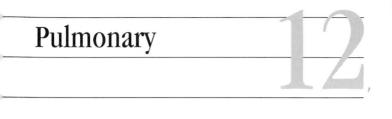

Pulmonary

Pulmonary disorders are among the most common causes of admission to an intensive care unit (ICU). The following formulas and facts are presented to aid in the diagnosis and management of patients presenting to the ICU with pulmonary conditions. Some of these formulas are not immediately useful in the clinical arena; however, they are of paramount importance in understanding normal and abnormal pulmonary physiology, and therefore cannot be excluded from this chapter.

I. **Lung volumes**   Normal values for pulmonary volumes and capacities in humans are depicted in Table 12–1:

Table 12–1.   Normal values for lung volumes in upright subjects

Volume or capacity	Approximate value in upright subjects
Total lung capacity (TLC)	6 L
Vital capacity (VC)	4.5 L
Residual volume (RV)	1.5 L
Inspiratory capacity (IC)	3 L
Functional residual capacity (FRC)	3 L
Inspiratory reserve volume (IRV)	2.5 L
Expiratory reserve volume (ERV)	1.5 L
Tidal volume (V_T)	0.5 L

The *vital capacity* (VC) is calculated as:

$$VC = IRV + ERV + V_T$$

The *residual volume* (RV) is calculated as the difference between the functional residual capacity (FRC) and the expiratory reserve volume (ERV):

$$RV = FRC - EV$$

Alternatively, if the total lung capacity (TLC) and vital capacity (VC) are known, the following formula can be utilized:

$$RV = TLC - VC$$

The oldest method to measure *FRC* is the *equilibration technique* according to the following formula:

$$FRC = [(C_1 \times V_1)/C_2] - V_1$$

where C_1 = known concentration of a test gas in the spirometer; V_1 = volume of gas in the spirometer; C_2 = the fractional value of the gas after the subject breathes in the spirometer until the concentration of the test gas equals that in the spirometer.

Another way to measure *FRC* is by the *nitrogen washout procedure* and the following formula:

$$FRC = (V_B \times C_B)/C_X$$

where V_B = amount of exhaled nitrogen volume in the bag; C_B = fractional concentration of nitrogen in the bag; C_X = subject initial fractional concentration of nitrogen (0.80).

Alternatively, FRC can be calculated using body plethysmography as:

$$FRC = (\Delta V/\Delta P)(P_B + \Delta P)$$

where ΔV = change in volume; ΔP = change in pressure; P_B = atmospheric pressure minus water vapor pressure (P_{H_2O}).

The *tidal volume* (V_T) is the sum of the dead space volume (V_D) and the alveolar volume (V_A):

$$V_T = V_D + V_A$$

The average *dead space volume* (V_D) is estimated as 1 mL/lb body weight. For an average 70-Kg man:

$$V_D = 70 \times 2.2 \times 1 = 154 \text{ mL}$$

II. Pulmonary ventilation: The easiest way of estimating *minute ventilation* ($\dot{V}_E$) is by the following formula:

$$\dot{V}_E = V_T \times RR = \text{mL/min}$$

where V_T = tidal volume; RR = respiratory rate.

Minute ventilation is also the sum of dead space (V_D) and alveolar ventilation ($\dot{V}_A$):

$$\dot{V}_E = \dot{V}_A + V_D$$

The *alveolar ventilation* ($\dot{V}_A$) can be calculated as:

$$\dot{V}_A = (V_T - V_D) \times N$$

where N = frequency of breathing in breaths per minute; V_D = dead space ventilation.

An alternative method requires knowledge of the CO_2 production by the patient. The *production of CO_2* (VCO_2) can be calculated as:

$$\dot{V}CO_2 = \dot{V}_A \times F_{ACO_2}$$

where F_{ACO_2} = fractional concentration of CO_2 in the alveolar gas; and

$$\dot{V}_A = \dot{V}CO_2 / F_{ACO_2}$$

Dead space ventilation ($\dot{V}_D$) can be calculated if the minute ventilation ($\dot{V}_E$) is known:

$$\dot{V}_D = \dot{V}_E \, ([Paco_2 - PEco_2])/Paco_2$$

The *partial pressure of alveolar CO_2* ($PACO_2$) is more convenient for these calculations and for practical purposes:

$$PACO_2 = F_{ACO_2} \times P_B$$

In normal lungs, the *arterial CO_2* ($Paco_2$) approximates the $PACO_2$. Therefore, the $\dot{V}_A$ formula can be rewritten as:

$$\dot{V}_A = K \, (Vco_2/Paco_2)$$

where K is a factor (0.863) that converts CO_2 concentrations to pressure (mm Hg).

III. Diffusion of gases: The rate of diffusion across a membrane is quantitatively expressed by *Fick's first law of diffusion*:

$$V = \frac{D \times A \times (P_1 - P_2)}{\Delta X}$$

where V = gas diffusion per unit time; D = diffusion constant for a particular gas; A = surface area of the membrane; $(P_1 - P_2)$ = partial pressure of the gas on either side of the membrane; ΔX = thickness of the membrane.

The *total resistance encountered by oxygen* ($1/D_L$) as it moves from the alveoli to combine with hemoglobin can be calculated by the following formula:

$$1/D_L = 1/D_M + 1/\theta Vc$$

where $1/D_M$ = membrane resistance; $1/\theta Vc$ = chemical reaction resistance.

The *diffusing capacity of a gas* (D_L) can be calculated as:

$$D_L = \frac{\dot{V}}{(P_A - P_C)} = \text{mL/min/mm Hg}$$

where $\dot{V}$ = the uptake of gas per minute; $(P_A - P_C)$ = mm Hg pressure difference of the gas.

For the *carbon monoxide diffusion capacity* (D_{LCO}), this generalized formula can be simplified to:

$$D_{LCO} = \frac{\dot{V}_{CO}}{P_{ACO}}$$

Because P_{CCO} remains near 0, it can usually be ignored in this equation.

IV. **Gas transport in blood:** The difference between the inspired and expired fractional concentration of oxygen represents the *oxygen uptake* ($\dot{V}O_2$):

$$\dot{V}O_2 = (\dot{V}_I \times F_IO_2) - (\dot{V}_E \times F_EO_2)$$

where $\dot{V}_I$ = volume of gas inhaled; F_IO_2 = fractional concentration of inspired oxygen; $\dot{V}_E$ = volume of gas exhaled; F_EO_2 = fractional concentration of expired oxygen.

The amount of *oxygen in solution in 100 mL of blood* is calculated as (assuming a partial oxygen pressure of 70 mm Hg):

$$(PO_2/760) \times \alpha O_2 = 70/760 \times 2.3 = 0.21 \text{ mL}/100 \text{ mL}$$

The PaO_2 at which hemoglobin is 50% saturated (P_{50}) can be calculated from the venous pH and arterial blood gases as:

$$P_{50} = \text{antilog} \frac{\text{Log } (1/k)}{n} = \text{normal 22–30 mm Hg}$$

where

$$(1/k) = (\text{antilog } [n \times \log PaO_{2_{7,4}}]) \times (100 - SaO_2/SaO_2)$$

$$\text{antilog } [n \times \log PaO_{2_{7,4}}] = \log PaO_2 - 0.5 (7.4 - \text{venous pH})$$

$$n = \text{Hill constant} = 2.7 \text{ for hemoglobin A}$$

The *Fick equation for oxygen consumption* ($\dot{V}O_2$) is calculated as:

$$\dot{V}O_2 = \dot{Q} (CaO_2 - C\overline{v}O_2)$$

where $\dot{Q}$ = cardiac output (L/min); CaO_2 = arterial oxygen content; $C\overline{v}O_2$ = mixed venous oxygen content.

The volume of carbon dioxide exhaled per unit time (*CO_2 production* or $\dot{V}CO_2$) is calculated as:

$$\dot{V}CO_2 = (\dot{V}_E \times F_ECO_2) - (\dot{V}_I \times F_ICO_2)$$

where $\dot{V}_E$ = volume of gas exhaled per unit time; F_ECO_2 = fractional concentration of carbon dioxide in the exhaled gas; V_I = volume of gas inhaled per unit time; F_ICO_2 = fractional concentration of inspired carbon dioxide.

Since the inspired gas usually contains negligible amounts of carbon dioxide, another representation of this formula is:

$$\dot{V}CO_2 = \dot{V}_E \times F_ECO_2$$

Another useful parameter in the characterization of tissue oxygenation is the *oxygen extraction ratio* (ERO_2), which is calculated with the following formula:

$$ERO_2 = \frac{\dot{V}O_2}{TO_2} = \frac{(CaO_2 - C\overline{v}O_2)}{CaO_2}$$

where TO_2 = systemic oxygen transport = $\dot{Q} \times CaO_2$ mL O_2/min

V. Pulmonary circulation: The *mean pulmonary artery pressure* ($\overline{PAP}$) can be calculated utilizing the following formula:

$$\overline{PAP} = (PVR \times PBF) + \overline{PAOP}$$

where PVR = pulmonary vascular resistance; PBF = pulmonary blood flow (which typically equals the cardiac output).

Reorganizing the above formula, the *pulmonary vascular resistance* (PVR) is then calculated as:

$$PVR = (\text{Mean PAP} - \overline{PAOP})/CO$$

where $\overline{PAOP}$ = pulmonary artery occlusion pressure; CO = cardiac output.

The pressures that surround the vessels in the pulmonary circulation contribute to the *transmural pressure* (Ptm) represented as:

$$Ptm = Pvas - Pis$$

where Pvas = vascular pressure; Pis = perivascular interstitial pressure.

When the left atrial pressure (Pla) is available, the *driving pressure* responsible for producing *pulmonary blood flow* is then calculated as:

$$(Ppa - Pla) = \dot{Q} \times Rvas$$

where Ppa = mean pulmonary arterial pressure; Pla = mean left atrial pressure; $\dot{Q}$ = pulmonary blood flow; Rvas = pulmonary vascular resistance.

The *pulmonary vascular compliance* (Cvas) can be calculated utilizing the following formula:

$$Cvas = \Delta Vvas/\Delta Pvas$$

where $\Delta Vvas$ = change in blood volume; $\Delta Pvas$ = change in vascular pressure.

The *blood flow zones* in an idealized upright lung with normal pressure differences are depicted in Table 12–2:

Table 12–2. Pulmonary blood flow zones

Blood flow zones	Pressures
I	Palv > Ppa > Ppv
II	Ppa > Palv > Ppv
III	Ppa > Ppv > Palv
IV	Ppa > Ppv > Palv

Palv = pressure surrounding the alveolar vessels; Ppa = mean pulmonary arterial pressure; Ppv = mean venous (left atrial) pressure.

VI. Mechanics and gas flow: The pressure inside the lungs relative to the pressure outside is known as the *transpulmonary pressure* (TP) and is calculated as:

$$TP = P_{alv} - P_{pl}$$

where P_{alv} = alveolar pressure; P_{pl} = pleural pressure

The change in volume (ΔV) for a unit pressure (ΔP) under conditions of no flow is the *static compliance*:

$$\text{Static compliance } (C_s) = \frac{\Delta V}{\Delta P}$$

Clinically, this formula can be simplified to:

$$C_s = \frac{V_T}{\text{Plateau airway pressure} - (\text{PEEP} + \text{autoPEEP})}$$

where V_T = tidal volume. Normal C_s value is 100 mL/cmH$_2$O.

The *dynamic compliance* (C_{dyn}) can be calculated by the following formula:

$$C_{dyn} = \frac{V_T}{\text{Peak airway pressure} - (\text{PEEP} + \text{autoPEEP})}$$

Normal C_{dyn} value is 100 mL/cmH$_2$O.

The *specific compliance* (C_{spec}) is calculated utilizing the following formula:

$$C_{spec} = C_s/\text{FRC}$$

The *chest wall compliance* (C_W) can be calculated as:

$$C_W = \frac{V_T}{\text{Airway pressure} - \text{Atmospheric pressure}}$$

Another formula that can be used under special circumstances (i.e., lung transplantation) is the *separate lung compliance* (C_X). This is calculated as:

$$C_X = \frac{V_T}{\text{Airway pressure} - \text{Intrapleural pressure}}$$

If the tidal volume, chest compliance, expiratory time, and expiratory resistance are known the *auto-PEEP* (AP) can be calculated by the formula:

$$AP = \frac{V_T}{C} \times \frac{1}{(e^{te/RxC} - 1)} - \text{PEEP}$$

where V_T = tidal volume; te = expiratory time; Rx = expiratory resistance; C = chest compliance.

The type of gas flow in the lung is *laminar flow* and is described mathematically by the *Poiseuille equation*:

$$\Delta P = \frac{8\mu l \dot{V}}{\pi r^4}$$

where ΔP = hydrostatic pressure drop; $\dot{V}$ = gas flow; μ = gas viscosity; l = path length; r = radius of the tube. From this equation, resistance (R = ΔP/V) can be calculated:

$$R = \frac{8\mu l}{\pi r^4}$$

On the other hand, *the pressure drop during turbulent flow* can be calculated utilizing the following formula:

$$\Delta P = \frac{l\mu^{1/4}\,\rho^{3/4}\,\dot{V}^{7/4}}{r^{19/4}}$$

where ΔP = pressure drop during turbulent flow; μ = viscosity; ρ = density.

The *Reynolds number* (Re) is the ratio of the pressure loss due to density-dependent or inertial flow versus the pressure loss due to viscous flow. This number is used to predict the nature of a particular flow and is calculated as:

$$Re = \frac{2\rho r\dot{V}}{\mu A}$$

The *airway resistance* (Raw) using body plethysmography can be calculated utilizing the following formula:

$$Raw = \frac{\Delta Vbox}{\dot{V}} \times \frac{Palv}{\Delta Vbox} = \frac{Palv}{\dot{V}}$$

where $\Delta Vbox$ = volume changes in the box; $\dot{V}$ = flow; $Palv$ = alveolar pressure.

The *work of the respiratory system* (W) can be calculated as:

$$W = P \times V$$

where P = pressure; V = volume.

VII. Ventilation/Perfusion: The physiologic *dead space* can be calculated utilizing the classic *Bohr equation*:

$$V_D/V_T = \frac{P_ACO_2 - P_{\bar{E}}CO_2}{P_ACO_2}$$

where P_ACO_2 = partial pressure of carbon dioxide in the alveolar gas; $P_{\bar{E}}CO_2$ = partial pressure of carbon dioxide in mixed expired gas.

The above formula with the *Enghoff modification* is used in clinical practice:

$$V_D/V_T = \frac{Paco_2 - P_{\bar{E}}CO_2}{Paco_2} = 0.30 \text{ in healthy subjects}$$

> 0.4 for intubated pt

The quantity of blood passing through pulmonary *right-to-left shunts* $(\dot{Q}s/\dot{Q})$ is calculated as:

$$\dot{Q}s/\dot{Q} = \frac{Cc'O_2 - CaO_2}{Cc'O_2 - C\bar{V}O_2}$$

where

$$Cc'O_2 = (Hb \times 1.38) + P_AO_2 \times \frac{\alpha}{760}$$

Therefore, the $\dot{Q}s/\dot{Q}$ formula can be rearranged as:

$$\dot{Q}s/\dot{Q} = \frac{(P_AO_2 - PaO_2) \times 0.0031}{(P_AO_2 - PaO_2) \times 0.0031 + (CaO_2 - C\bar{v}O_2)}$$

VIII. Alveolar gas equation: The *alveolar air equation* is based firmly on Dalton's law, but is expressed in terms that emphasize alveolar O_2 and CO_2:

$$P_AO_2 = (P_{ATM} - P_{H_2O}) FiO_2 - PCO_2/RQ$$

where P_AO_2 = partial pressure of O_2 in the alveolus under present conditions; P_{ATM} = current, local atmospheric pressure. P_{H_2O} = vapor pressure of water at body temperature and 100 percent relative humidity; FiO_2 = fraction of inspired O_2; PCO_2 = partial pressure of CO_2 in arterial blood; RQ = respiratory quotient.

At *sea level*, this equation can be simplified to:

$$P_AO_2 = 150 - 1.25 \times Paco_2$$

The *arterial oxygen tension (PaO₂) corrected for age* is calculated as:

$$PaO_2 \text{ age-corrected} = 100 - 1/3 \text{ age (in years)}$$

The *alveolar-arterial oxygen gradient* is *age-corrected* according to the following formula:

$$\text{Age correction} = 2.5 + (0.25 \times [\text{age in years}])$$

IX. Pulmonary fluid exchange: The *pulmonary capillary pressure* (Ppc) can be calculated utilizing the following formula:

$$Ppc = Pla + (r_v/r_t) (Ppa - Pla)$$

where Pla = left atrial pressure; r_v/r_t = total vascular resistance; Ppa − Pla = pressure gradient across the pulmonary circulation.

The following equation can be used to approximate the colloid *osmotic pressure of plasma* (Π_P):

$$\Pi_P = 2.1\, C_P + 0.16\, C_P^2$$

where C_P = serum protein concentration.

The concentration of protein in the tissues (C_T) relative to plasma (C_P) can be calculated as:

$$C_T/C_P = \frac{(1 - \theta d)\, Jv}{Jv} + \frac{PS\,(C_P - C_T)}{Jv\, C_P}$$

where θd = osmotic reflection coefficient (solute selectivity of the pulmonary capillary wall); C_P = protein concentration of plasma; Jv = capillary filtration; PS = permeability coefficient times the surface area for exchange.

The movement of fluid across the capillary can be represented utilizing the *Starling relationship*:

$$Jv = \text{filtration pressure} - \text{absorption pressure}$$

$$Jv = Kfc \, [(Ppc - P_T) - \theta d \, (\Pi_P - \Pi_T)]$$

where Kfc = solvent permeability of the pulmonary capillary wall.

The *normal pressures in the pulmonary capillary endothelium* are depicted in Table 12–3:

Table 12–3. Normal capillary endothelium filtration pressures

Parameter	Normal value
Ppc	7 mm Hg
P_T	−5 mm Hg
Π_P	28 mm Hg
Π_T	17 mm Hg
Kfc	0.02 mL/min/100g/mm Hg
θd	1

Ppc = capillary pressure; P_T = interstitial hydrostatic fluid pressure; Π_P = plasma colloid-osmotic pressure; Π_T = tissue colloid-osmotic pressure; Kfc = solvent permeability of the pulmonary capillary wall; θd = solute selectivity of the pulmonary capillary wall.

X. Ventilator weaning: Some of the standard indices predicting weaning success are depicted in Table 12–4:

Table 12–4. Standard indices for weaning success

Index	Value suggesting success
Minute ventilation ($\dot{V}_E$)	< 10 L/min
Tidal volume (V_T)	5 mL/Kg
Vital capacity (V_C)	$2 \times V_T$
Maximal voluntary ventilation (MVV)	$2 \times \dot{V}_E$

Another commonly employed weaning index is the *rapid shallow breathing index* (RSBI), which is calculated as:

$$RSBI = f/V_T$$

where f = frequency; V_T = tidal volume. Successful weaning is usually accomplished if the RSBI is <100 breaths/min/L.

The *CROP* (acronym for compliance, rate, oxygenation, and pressure) index is an integrative index and is calculated with the following formula:

$$CROP \text{ index} = (C_{dyn} \times P_I\text{max} \times [Pao_2/P_AO_2])/rate$$

where C_{dyn} = dynamic compliance; P_imax = maximal inspiratory pressure. Weaning success occurs if value is ≥ 13 mL/breath/min.

   XI. Acid-base formulas: The reader is encouraged to also refer to the formulas and facts depicted in Chapter 13 of this handbook.

   The hydrogen ion concentration expressed in terms of *pH* is calculated as:

$$pH = -\log [H^+]$$

Using the *Henderson-Hasselbach equation* the pH is then calculated as:

$$pH = pK + \log \frac{[HCO_3^-]}{[CO_2]}$$

This equation can be applied clinically by modifying the formula as follows:

$$pH = 6.1 + \log \frac{[HCO_3^-]}{0.03 \, P_{CO_2}}$$

For *acute respiratory acidosis or alkalosis* the pH appropriate for acute in Pa_{CO_2}:

$$\Delta \, pH \, (\text{from } 7.40) = \Delta Pa_{CO_2} \, (\text{from } 40 \text{ mm Hg}) \times 0.007$$

The bicarbonate level appropriate for change in Pa_{CO_2} is calculated in *acute respiratory alkalosis*:

$$\text{Fall in } HCO_3^- \, (\text{from } 24 \text{ mmol/L}) = 1 \text{ to } 3 \, (\Delta \, Pa_{CO_2}/10)$$

The bicarbonate level appropriate for change in Pa_{CO_2} is calculated in *chronic respiratory alkalosis*:

$$\text{Fall in } HCO_3^- \, (\text{from } 24 \text{ mmol/L}) = 2 \text{ to } 5 \, (\Delta \, Pa_{CO_2}/10)$$

The bicarbonate level appropriate for change in Pa_{CO_2} is calculated in *acute respiratory acidosis*:

$$\text{Rise in } HCO_3^- = (\Delta Pa_{CO_2}/10) \pm 3$$

The bicarbonate level appropriate for change in Pa_{CO_2} is calculated in *chronic respiratory acidosis*:

$$\text{Rise in } HCO_3^- = (\Delta Pa_{CO_2} \times 4)/10 \pm 4$$

The compensatory *change in Pa_{CO_2}* for the degree of *metabolic acidosis* as expressed by a drop in bicarbonate is calculated as:

$$\text{Drop in } Pa_{CO_2} = 1 \text{ to } 1.5 \times \Delta HCO_3^-$$

The compensatory *change in Pa_{CO_2}* for the degree of *metabolic alkalosis* as expressed by a rise in bicarbonate is calculated as:

$$\Delta Pa_{CO_2} = 0.25 \text{ to } 1.0 \times \Delta HCO_3^- \, (\text{from } 24 \text{ mmol/L})$$

To calculate the *bicarbonate deficit (BD) in metabolic acidosis*, the following formula is commonly employed:

$$BD = 0.5 \times (weight\ in\ Kg) \times \Delta HCO_3^- \ (from\ 24\ mmol/L)$$

If the *pH is less than 7.1*, the formula is modified to:

$$BD = 0.8 \times (weight\ in\ Kg) \times \Delta HCO_3^- \ (from\ 24\ mmol/L)$$

The *anion gap* (AG) is calculated as:

$$AG = ([Na^+] + [K^+]) - ([Cl^-] + [HCO_3^-])$$

$$AG\ normal = 8 - 12\ mEq(mmol)/L$$

XII. Other facts and formulas: The approximate alveolar PO_2 at different atmospheres during *hyperbaric oxygen therapy* (HBO) is depicted in Table 12–5:

Table 12–5. Effects of hyperbaric oxygen therapy at different environmental pressures on the alveolar PO_2

Environmental pressure (atmospheres)	Environmental pressure (mm hg)	Alveolar PO_2 breathing air (21% oxygen)
1	760	102
2	1520	262
3	2280	422
6	4560	902

Renal and
Fluid–Electrolytes

Fluid and electrolyte balance is a challenging area of critical care. In addition, renal problems are common, and their management incorporates a number of useful formulas and facts.

I. Acid-base equations/facts: The normal relationship between bicarbonate (HCO_3^-), hydrogen ions (H^+) and carbon dioxide is expressed in the *Henderson equation*:

$$[H^+] = 24 \times (P_{CO_2}/[HCO_3^-])$$

where P_{CO_2} = partial pressure of carbon dioxide.

This interaction can also be represented by the *Henderson-Hasselbalch equation*:

$$pH = 6.10 + \log ([HCO_3^-]/0.03 \times P_{CO_2})$$

The mean response equations for simple acid-base disturbances are depicted in Table 13–1:

Table 13–1. Selected response equations for simple acid-base disturbances

Acid-base disturbance	Equation
Metabolic acidosis	$\Delta P_{aCO_2} \approx 1.2 \ \Delta[HCO_3^-]$
Metabolic alkalosis	$\Delta P_{aCO_2} \approx 0.7 \ \Delta[HCO_3^-]$
Respiratory acidosis	
Acute	$\Delta[HCO_3^-] \approx 0.1 \ \Delta P_{aCO_2}$
	$\Delta[H^+] \approx 0.75 \ \Delta P_{aCO_2}$
Chronic	$\Delta[HCO_3^-] \approx 0.3 \ \Delta P_{aCO_2}$
	$\Delta[H^+] \approx 0.3 \ \Delta P_{aCO_2}$
Respiratory alkalosis	
Acute	$\Delta[HCO_3^-] \approx 0.2 \ \Delta P_{aCO_2}$
	$\Delta[H^-] \approx 0.75 \ \Delta P_{aCO_2}$
Chronic	$\Delta[HCO_3^-] \approx 0.5 \ \Delta P_{aCO_2}$
	$\Delta[H^+] \approx 0.5 \ \Delta P_{aCO_2}$

The amount of *NaHCO₃ needed* to raise the serum [HCO₃⁻] can be calculated as:

$$\text{NaHCO}_3 \text{ required (mEq)} = \text{Body weight (Kg)} \times 0.7$$
$$\times \text{ (Desired [HCO}_3^-] - \text{Current [HCO}_3^-]$$

Alternatively, the following formula can be utilized to calculate the *base deficit* in metabolic acidosis:

$$\text{HCO}_3^- \text{ deficit} = (\text{desired HCO}_3 - \text{observed HCO}_3)$$
$$\times .4 \text{ (body weight (Kg))}$$

The *chloride deficit* in the treatment of metabolic alkalosis can be calculated by the following formula:

$$\text{Cl}^- \text{ Deficit (mEq)} = 0.5 \text{ (weight in Kg)}(103 - \text{measured Cl}^-)$$

II. **Renal function formulas:** The normal *glomerular filtration rate* (GFR) can be approximated, adjusted for age, based on the following formulas:

$$\text{Before 45 years:} \qquad \text{GFR} = 12.49 - 0.37 \text{ (age)}$$
$$\text{At or above 45 years: GFR} = 153 - 1.07 \text{ (age)}$$

A formula derived by *Cockcroft and Gault* is commonly used to estimate *creatinine clearance*:

$$\text{Creatinine clearance (mL/min)} = \frac{140 - \text{age}}{\text{Serum creatinine (mg/dl)}} \times \frac{\text{Body weight (Kg)}}{72}$$

In women, the value obtained from this equation is multiplied by a factor of 0.85.

This formula can also be adjusted for lean body weight (LBW) calculated from:

$$\text{LBW (male)} = 50 \text{ Kg} + 2.3 \text{ Kg/inch} > 5 \text{ feet}$$

$$\text{LBW (female)} = 45.5 \text{ Kg} + 2.3 \text{ Kg/inch} > 5 \text{ feet}$$

Alternatively, the creatinine clearance (C_{cr}) can be measured as:

$$C_{cr} = \frac{(U_{cr} \cdot V)}{P_{cr}}$$

where U_{cr} = concentration of creatinine in a timed collection of urine; P_{cr} = concentration of creatinine in the plasma; V = urine flow rate (volume divided by period of collection).

Another method commonly employed to calculate the creatinine clearance is *Jelliffe's formula*:

$$C_{cr} = \frac{98 - 0.8 \text{ (age } -20)}{P_{cr}}$$

In this formula, age is rounded to nearest decade. In females, the above result is multiplied by a factor of 0.9.

A more complicated and potentially more accurate way to calculate creatinine clearance is *Mawer's formula*:

$$C_{cr} \text{ (males)} = \frac{\text{LBW } [29.3 - (0.203 \times \text{age})][1 - (0.03 \times P_{cr})]}{14.4 \; (P_{cr})}$$

$$C_{cr} \text{ (females)} = \frac{\text{LBW } [25.3 - (0.174 \times \text{age})][1 \; (0.03 \times P_{cr})]}{14.4 \; (P_{cr})}$$

Hull's formula for creatinine clearance is calculated as:

$$C_{cr} = [(145 - \text{age})/P_{cr}] - 3$$

In females, the result is multiplied by a factor of 0.85.

Ranges for *creatinine clearance* under selected conditions are depicted in Table 13–2:

Table 13–2. Creatinine clearance values under selected conditions

Condition	Value
Normal	> 100 mL/min
Mild renal failure	40–60 mL/min
Moderate renal failure	10–40 mL/min
Severe renal failure	< 10 mL/min

III. **Selected electrolytes:** The *transtubular potassium gradient* (TTKG) allows one to estimate the potassium secretory response in the cortical collecting duct. This index corrects for water reabsorption in the cortical and medullary collecting ducts:

$$\text{TTKG} = \text{Corrected urine } K^+/\text{Serum } K^+$$

$$\text{Corrected urine } K^+ = \frac{\text{Urine } K^+}{U_{osm}/P_{osm}}$$

The normal renal conservation of potassium is reflected by a TTKG < 2.

The percentage of *magnesium retention* (MR) can be calculated by the following formula:

$$\text{MR } (\%) = 1 - \frac{\begin{array}{c}\text{Postinfusion} \\ \text{24-h} \\ \text{urine Mg}\end{array} - \left(\begin{array}{c}\text{(Preinfusion} \\ \text{urine Mg/Cr ratio}\end{array} \times \begin{array}{c}\text{Postinfusion)} \\ \text{urine Cr}\end{array}\right)}{\text{Total elemental magnesium infused}} \times 100$$

The *fractional tubular reabsorption of phosphate* (TRP) allows for quantification of renal phosphate wasting and is calculated as:

$$\text{TRP} = 1 - C_{PO4}/C_{cr}$$

where C_{PO4}/C_{cr} = fractional excretion of phosphate.

In conditions such as proximal renal tubular acidosis, the *fractional excretion of HCO_3^-* (FEHCO$_3^-$) can be calculated as:

$$\text{FEHCO}_3^- = \frac{\text{Urine [HCO}_3^-] \text{ (mEq/L)}}{\text{Serum [HCO}_3^-] \text{ (mEq/L)}} \times \frac{\text{Serum creatinine (mg/dL)}}{\text{Urine creatinine (mg/dL)}} \times 100$$

The *correction of calcium* based on the serum albumin/globulin levels is calculated as:

$$\% \text{ Ca bound} = 8 \text{ (albumin)} + 2 \text{ (globulin)} + 3$$

Another formula to correct *calcium based on total protein* is:

$$\text{Corrected Ca} = \text{measured Ca}/(0.6 + (\text{total protein}/8.5))$$

A quick bedside formula for calculation of the corrected calcium:

$$\text{Corrected Ca} = \text{Calcium} - \text{albumin} + 4$$

IV. Osmolality formulas: To calculate the *serum osmolality* (Osm) the following formula is employed:

$$\text{Osm} = 2\text{Na}^+ + \text{BUN (mg/dL)}/2.8 + \text{glucose (mg/dL)}/18$$

The *osmolar gap* (OG) is calculated as the difference between the measured osmolality and the calculated osmolality:

$$\text{OG} = \text{Measured osmolality} - \text{Calculated osmolality}$$

The approximate *urine osmolality* can be calculated from the formula:

$$\text{mOsm} \sim (\text{Urine specific gravity} - 1) \times 40,000$$

V. Water balance: To estimate the amount of *total body water* (TBW), the following formula is frequently employed:

$$\text{TBW} = \text{Body weight (Kg)} \times 60\%$$

The *water deficit* of a patient can be estimated by the following equation:

$$\text{Water deficit} = 0.6 \times \text{Body weight in Kg} \times (\text{PNa}/140 - 1)$$

where PNa = plasma sodium concentration.

Alternatively the *free water deficit* from the osmolality can be calculated as:

$$\text{H}_2\text{O deficit (L)} = \text{Total body weight (Kg)} \times .6 \left(1 - \frac{\text{normal osm}}{\text{observed osm}}\right)$$

To calculate the *free water clearance* based on the osmolar clearance, the following formula can be utilized:

$$\text{Free water clearance} = \text{Urine volume} - \text{Osmolar clearance}$$

where the *osmolar clearance* is calculated as:

$$\text{Osmolar clearance} = \frac{\text{Urine osmolarity} \times \text{urine volume}}{\text{Plasma osmolality}}$$

The *excess water* (EW) of a patient is calculated as:

$$EW = TBW - [\text{Actual plasma Na/Desired plasma Na}] \times TBW$$

VI. **Urinary/Renal indices:** The most common *urinary indices* used in the differential diagnosis of acute renal failure are depicted in Table 13–3:

Table 13–3. Commonly used urinary indices in acute renal failure

Index	Prerenal	Acute tubular necrosis
Specific gravity	>1.020	<1.010
Urinary osmolality ($mOsm/Kg\ H_2O$)	>500	<350
U_{osm}/P_{osm}	>1.3	<1.1
Urinary Na^+ (mEq/L)	<20	>40
U/P Cr	>40	<20
RFI	<1	>1
FENa(%)	<1	>1

Cr = creatinine; P = plasma; RFI = renal failure index; U = urine; FENa = fractional excretion of sodium.

To calculate the *renal failure index* (RFI) the following formula is commonly employed:

$$RFI = \frac{U\ Na}{U/P\ Cr}$$

The *fractional excretion of sodium* (FENa) is calculated as:

$$FENa\ (\%) = \frac{\text{Quantity of } Na^+ \text{ excreted}}{\text{Quantity of } Na^+ \text{ filtered}} \times 100$$

or

$$FENa\ (\%) = \frac{U/P\ Na^+ \times 100}{U/P\ Cr}$$

or

$$FENa\ (\%) = \frac{U_{Na} \times V}{P_{Na} \times (U_{Cr} \times V/P_{Cr})} \times 100$$

or

$$FENa\ (\%) = \frac{U_{Na} \times P_{Cr}}{P_{Na} \times U_{Cr}} \times 100$$

where U_{Na} = urine sodium concentration; V = urine flow rate; P_{Na} = plasma sodium concentration; U_{Cr} = urine creatinine concentration; P_{Cr} = plasma creatinine concentration.

VII. Hemodialysis formulas: The following equations are useful in the management of the chronic hemodialysis patient.

The *protein catabolic rate* (PCR) is calculated as:

$$PCR \ (g/Kg/day) = 0.22 + \frac{0.036 \times ID \ BUN \times 24}{ID \ interval}$$

where ID BUN = interdialytic rise in blood urea nitrogen (BUN) in mg/dL; ID interval = interdialytic interval in hours.

Alternatively, if blood urea is measured the PCR can be calculated utilizing the following formula:

$$PCR \ (g/Kg/day) = 0.22 + \frac{0.1 \times ID \ urea \times 24}{ID \ interval}$$

where ID urea = interdialytic rise in blood urea in mmol/L.

If the patient has a significant urine output, the contribution of the urinary urea excretion must be added to the PCR calculation and is calculated as:

$$Urine \ contribution \ to \ PCR = \frac{Urine \ urea \ N \ (g) \times 150}{ID \ interval \ (hr) \times Body \ weight \ (Kg)}$$

Alternatively, if urine urea is measured:

$$Urine \ contribution \ to \ PCR = \frac{Urine \ urea \ (mmol) \times 4.2}{ID \ interval \ (hr) \times Body \ weight \ (Kg)}$$

To calculate the *percentage of recirculation* during hemodialysis, the following formula is utilized:

$$\% \ Recirculation = \frac{A2 - A1}{A2 - V} \times 100$$

where A2 = blood urea or creatinine concentration in arterial blood line after blood pump is stopped; A1 = arterial line blood urea or creatinine concentration; V = venous line urea or creatinine concentration.

The *volume of distribution of urea* can be calculated as follows:

Males: $V = 2.447 - 0.09516A + 0.1074H + 0.3362W$

Females: $V = -2.097 + 0.1069H + 0.2466W$

where V = volume in liters; A = age in years; H = height in centimeters; W = weight in kilograms.

The calculation of *residual renal function* for dialysis three times per week:

$$GFR = \frac{V \times U}{t \times (0.25 \ U_1 + 0.75 \ U_2)}$$

where V = urine volume in interdialytic period; U = urine urea nitrogen or urea concentration; t = interdialytic period in minutes; U_1 = postdialysis BUN or blood urea on first dialysis of the week; U_2 = predialysis BUN or blood urea on second dialysis of the week.

The *percent reduction of urea* (PRU) can be calculated utilizing the following formula:

$$PRU = \frac{\text{Pre-urea} - \text{Post-urea}}{\text{Pre-urea}} \times 100$$

The *urea reduction ratio* (URR) is calculated as:

$$URR = 100 \times \left(1 - \frac{\text{Post-urea}}{\text{Pre-urea}}\right)$$

VIII. **Urinalysis:** Please refer also to Chapter 18 for additional laboratory values. The most common *urinalysis* manifestations of renal diseases are depicted in Table 13–4:

Table 13–4. Urinalysis in different conditions

Condition	Findings	
Prerenal failure	SG:	>1.015
	pH:	<6
	Prot:	trace to 1+
	Sed:	sparse hyaline, fine granular cases or bland
Postrenal failure	SG:	1.010
	pH:	>6
	Prot:	trace to 1+
	Hb:	+
	Sed:	RBCs, WBCs
Acute tubular necrosis (ATN)	"Muddy" brown urine	
	SG:	1.010
	pH:	6–7
	Prot:	trace to 1+
	Blood:	+
	Sed:	RBCs, WBCs, RTE cells, RTE casts, pigmented casts
Glomerular diseases	SG:	>1.020
	pH:	>6
	Prot:	1 to 4+
	Sed:	RBCs, RBC casts, WBC, oval fat bodies, free fat droplets, fatty casts
Vascular diseases	SG:	>1.020 if proglomerular
	pH:	<6
	Prot:	trace to 2+
	Sed:	RBCs and RBC casts with glomerular involvement
Interstitial diseases	SG:	1.010
	pH:	6–7
	Prot:	trace to 1+
	Sed:	WBCs, WBC casts, eosinophils, RBCs, RTE cells

RBC = red blood cells; RTE = renal tubular epithelial cells; WBC = white blood cells;
SG = urine specific gravity; Prot = protein; Sed = urinary sediment.

Some elements and substances can modify the color of urine in humans as depicted in Table 13–5:

Table 13–5. Urine color based on the presence of elements or substances

Elements/Substances	Characteristic color
White blood cells	Milky white
Precipitated phosphates	
Chyle	
Bilirubin	Yellow/amber
Chloroquine	
Sulfasalazine	
Nitrofurantoin	
Urobilin	
Phenazopyridine	Brown/red
Hemoglobin	
Myoglobin	
Red blood cells	
Phenothiazines	
Phenytoin	
Porphyrins	
Beets	
Red-colored candies	
Melanin	Brown/black
Phenol	
Methyldopa	
Metronidazole	
Quinine	
Pseudomonas infection	Blue/green
Amitriptyline	
Methylene blue	
Biliverdin	
Propofol	

IX. **Other formulas/facts:** To determine whether a patient has aminoaciduria or not the *fractional reabsorption of an amino acid* (FR_A) is determined utilizing the following formula:

$$FR_A = 1 - [Urine]_A/[Plasma]_A \div [Urine]_{Cr}/[Plasm]_{Cr} \times 100\%$$

The normal *urinary excretion of amino acids* in patients older than 2 years is depicted in Table 13–6:

Table 13–6. Normal urinary excretion of selected amino acids

Amino acid	Normal excretion (mg/g creatinine)
Cystine	18
Lysine	130
Arginine	16
Ornithine	22

When acute renal failure (ARF) is due to *uric acid nephropathy* (UAN), the following equation is generally > 1:

$$\text{Index} = \frac{\text{spot urine uric acid (mg/dL)}}{\text{spot urine creatinine (mg/dL)}} = {>}1.0$$

Statistics and Epidemiology

Although not commonly considered a clinical subject, statistics and epidemiology form the cornerstone of clinical practice. An understanding of statistical principles is necessary to comprehend the published literature and to practice in a rational manner. The purpose of this chapter is to review some of the basic statistical principles and formulas. More in-depth discussion can be obtained in texts of biostatistics.

1. **Measurements of disease frequency:** *Prevalence* is the most frequently used measure of disease frequency and is defined as:

$$\text{Prevalence} = \frac{\text{Number of existing cases of a disease}}{\text{Total population at a given point in time}}$$

Incidence quantifies the number of **new** cases that develop in a population at risk during a specific time interval:

$$\text{Cumulative incidence} = \frac{\text{Number of new cases of a disease during a given time period}}{\text{Total population at risk}}$$

Cumulative incidence (CI) reflects the probability that an individual develops a disease during a given time period. *Incidence density* (ID) allows one to account for varying periods of follow-up and is calculated as:

$$\text{ID} = \frac{\text{New cases of the disease during a given period of time}}{\text{Total person-time of observation}}$$

Special types of incidence and prevalence measures are reported. *Mortality rate* is an incidence measure:

$$\text{Mortality rate} = \frac{\text{Number of deaths}}{\text{Total population}}$$

Case-fatality rate is another incidence measure:

$$\text{Case-fatality rate} = \frac{\text{Number of deaths from the disease}}{\text{Number of cases of the disease}}$$

Attack rate is also an incidence measure:

$$\text{Attack rate} = \frac{\text{Number of cases of the disease}}{\text{Total population at risk for a given time period}}$$

2. **Laboratory testing:** The performance of a laboratory test is commonly reported in terms of sensitivity and specificity defined as:

$$\text{Sensitivity} = \frac{\text{True-positives}}{\text{True-positives} + \text{false-negatives}}$$

$$\text{Specificity} = \frac{\text{True-negatives}}{\text{True-negatives} + \text{false-positives}}$$

Thus, *sensitivity* measures the number of people who truly have the disease who test positive. *Specificity* measures the number of people who do not have the disease who test negative.

These crude measurements of laboratory performance do not take into account the level at which a test is determined to be positive. *Receiver operator characteristics curves (ROC curves)* examine the performance of a test throughout its range of values. An area under the ROC curve of 1.0 is a perfect test, whereas a test that is no better than flipping a coin has an area under the ROC curve of 0.5.

As clinicians examining a positive test, we are most interested in determining whether a patient actually has the disease. The *positive predictive value (PPV)* provides this probability:

$$\text{PPV} = \frac{\text{True-positives}}{\text{True-positives} + \text{false-positives}}$$

$$\text{PPV} = \frac{\text{Prevalence} \times \text{sensitivity}}{\text{Prevalence} \times \text{sensitivity} + (1 - \text{prevalence}) \times (1 - \text{specificity})}$$

Negative predictive value (NPV) describes the probability of a patient's testing negative for a disease who does not have that disease:

$$\text{NPV} = \frac{\text{True-negatives}}{\text{True-negatives} + \text{false-negatives}}$$

$$\text{NPV} = \frac{(1 - \text{prevalence}) \times \text{specificity}}{(1 - \text{prevalence}) \times \text{specificity} + \text{prevalence} \times (1 - \text{sensitivity})}$$

3. **Describing data:** A large collection of data cannot really be appreciated by simple scrutiny. Summary or descriptive statistics help to describe the data succinctly. Two measures are usually employed: a measure of central tendency and a measure of dispersion.

Measures of central tendency include mean, median and mode. *Mean* is the common arithmetical average:

$$\text{Mean} = \sum_{i=1}^{n} X_i/n$$

Median is the middle value. The value such that one-half of the data points fall below and one-half fall above. *Mode* is the most frequently occurring data point.

Measures of dispersion include the range, interquartile range, variance, and standard deviation.

$$\text{Range} = \text{Greatest value} - \text{Least value}$$

The *interquartile range (IQR)* is the range of the middle 50 percent of the data.

$$\text{IQR} = U_{75} - L_{25}$$

where U_{75} is the upper 75th percentile and L_{25} is the lower 25th percentile. *Sample variance* is the average of the squared distances between each of the values and the mean:

$$\text{Sample variance } (s^2) = \frac{\Sigma \, (x - \bar{x})^2}{n - 1}$$

Standard deviation is the square root of this value:

$$\text{Standard deviation}(s) = \sqrt{\frac{\Sigma \, (x - \bar{x})^2}{n - 1}}$$

4. **Statistical testing:** *Hypothesis testing* involves conducting a test of statistical significance, quantifying the degree to which random variability may account for the observed results. In performing hypothesis testing two types of error can be made (Table 14–1).

Table 14–1. Four possible outcomes of hypothesis testing

Conclusion of the test	Null hypothesis true	Alternative hypothesis true
Do not reject null hypothesis (not statistically significant)	Correct result	Type II error
Reject null hypothesis (statistically significant)	Type I error	Correct result

Type I errors refer to a situation in which statistical significance is found when no difference actually exists. The probability of making a Type I error is equal to the *p* values of a statistical test and is commonly represented by the Greek letter α. Traditionally, α levels of 0.05 are used for statistical significance. *Type II errors* refer to failure to declare that a difference exists when there is a real difference between the study groups. The probability of making a Type II error is represented by the Greek letter β. The *power* of a test is calculated as $1 - \beta$ and is the probability of declaring a statistically significant difference if one truly exists.

5. Statistical methods: The following formulas and methods are the most frequently used test for biologic data.

Chi-square test (χ^2) is used for discrete data such as counts. The general form of a chi-square test is:

$$\chi^2 = \sum \frac{(\text{Observed} - \text{expected})^2}{\text{Expected}}$$

Chi-square testing is commonly used in contingency tables (Table 14–2).

Table 14–2.   Contingency table

	Diseased	Not diseased	Totals
Exposed	a	b	a + b
Not exposed	c	d	c + d
	a + c	b + d	a + b + c + d

Where the expected frequencies for each cell of the contingency table is the product of the marginal totals divided by the grand total (Table 14–3).

Table 14–3.   Table of expected values

	Diseased	Not diseased	Totals
Exposed	$\dfrac{(a + c)(a + b)}{a + b + c + d}$	$\dfrac{(b + d)(a + b)}{a + b + c + d}$	
Not exposed	$\dfrac{(a + c)(c + d)}{a + b + c + d}$	$\dfrac{(b + d)(c + d)}{a + b + c + d}$	

Yates correction: When the expected value of any particular cell is less than 5, the Yates correction is used. This is calculated as:

$$\chi^2 \; Yates \; corrected = \sum \frac{(|\text{Observed} - \text{expected}| - 0.5)^2}{\text{Expected}}$$

Relative risk: The data within a contingency table are commonly summarized in measures such as the relative risk. If we gather groups based on their exposure status, relative risk can be calculated as:

$$Relative \; risk = \frac{\dfrac{a}{a + b}}{\dfrac{c}{c + d}}$$

This figure represents the risk of becoming diseased if you are exposed (a/a + b) divided by the risk if you are not exposed (c/c + d), which is why it is called relative risk. If the relative risk is calculated at 4.0, then the risk of becoming diseased if you are exposed is four times that of people who are not exposed.

Odds ratio: If we gather groups based on disease status, the odds ratio is calculated as an approximation to the relative risk:

$$Odds\ ratio = \frac{\dfrac{a}{b}}{\dfrac{c}{d}}$$

This measure is the ratio of the odds of getting disease if you are exposed and the odds of becoming diseased if you are not.

t-test: Usually used in comparing means:

$$2\ sample\ independent\ t\text{-}test = \frac{\bar{x}_1 - \bar{x}_2}{S_p \sqrt{\dfrac{1}{n_1} + \dfrac{1}{n_2}}}$$

with $(n_1 - 1) + (n_2 - 1)$ degrees of freedom, where:

$$S_p = \frac{\sum (x_1 - \bar{x}_1)^2 + \sum (x_2 - \bar{x}_2)^2}{(n_1 - 1) + (n_2 - 1)}$$

$$Paired\ t\text{-}test = \frac{\text{Mean difference of the pairs}}{SD \left(\sqrt{\dfrac{1}{n}} \right)}$$

with $n - 1$ degrees of freedom

Normal approximation for comparing two proportions: A method for comparing whether two proportions are significantly different:

$$z = \frac{P_1 - P_2}{\sqrt{\dfrac{(P_1 \times [1 - P_1])}{n_1} + \dfrac{(P_2 \times [1 - P_2])}{n_2}}}$$

Analysis of variance: This method is commonly used to compare means across more than two categories.

Regression techniques: Generally obtained via computer programs; can be used to predict a continuous variable from single or multiple regressors which are categorical, continuous, or both.

15 Toxicology

Toxic ingestions and intoxications are common reasons for admission to the intensive care unit. The following formulas, facts, and laboratory values may help the critical care practitioner diagnose and manage these patients.

1. Basic formulas: The *therapeutic index* (TI) of a drug can be calculated as:

$$TI = \frac{LD50}{ED50}$$

where LD50 = median lethal dose; ED50 = median effective dose.

The *margin of safety* (MS) of a drug uses the ED99 for the desired effect and the LD1 for the undesired effect:

$$MS = \frac{LD1}{ED99}$$

The *apparent volume of distribution* (V_d) can be calculated by the following equation:

$$V_d = \frac{Dose_{iv}}{C_0}$$

where $Dose_{iv}$ = the intravenous dose; C_0 = the extrapolated plasma concentration at time zero.

For those agents that follow a two-compartment model, the following formula is used to assess the *volume of the central compartment* (V_c):

$$V_c = \frac{Dose_{iv}}{A + B}$$

where A and B represent disposition constants of a two-compartment model. In addition, the *peripheral compartment* (V_p) can be calculated as:

$$V_p = \frac{Dose_{iv}}{B}$$

where B is derived from the elimination or equilibrium phase of a two-compartment model.

The *total body clearance* (CI) of a drug can be calculated as the sum of clearances by individual organs:

$$Cl = Cl_r + Cl_h + Cl_i + \ .....$$

where Cl_r = renal clearance; Cl_h = hepatic clearance; Cl_i = intestinal clearance.

2. **Osmolality formulas:** To calculate *serum osmolality* the following formula is usually applied:

$$Calc. \ Osmolality \ (mOsm/Kg) = 2Na + BUN/2.8 + Glucose/18$$

The *osmolal gap* (OG) is useful in several intoxications and is calculated as:

$$OG = Measured \ osmolality - calculated \ osmolality$$

To calculate the contribution to measured osmolality of alcohols (also known as *osmol ratios*), the alcohol concentration (mg/dL) is divided by the numbers depicted in Table 15–1:

Table 15–1. Osmolal ratios of different alcohols

Ethanol	Ethylene glycol	Isopropanol	Methanol
4.6	6.2	6.0	3.2

3. **Digitalis intoxication:** In order to treat digitalis (digoxin or digitoxin) poisoning appropriately it is important to assess the *digitalis body load:*

$$Body \ load \ (mg) = (serum \ digoxin \ concentration) \times 5.6$$
$$\times \ (body \ weight \ in \ Kg) \div 1000$$

The *dose of digitalis antibodies* (Digibind®) is determined by dividing the body load by 0.6 mg/vial:

$$Dose \ (number \ of \ vials) = Body \ load \ (mg) \div 0.6 \ (mg/vial)$$

4. **Miscellaneous:** The *Rumack-Matthew nomogram* for acetaminophen poisoning is depicted in Figure 15–1:

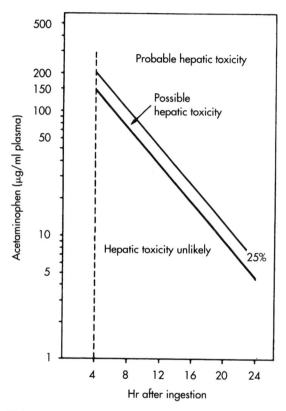

Figure 15–1.
Rumack-Matthew nomogram for acetaminophen poisoning. (From Rumack BH, Matthew H: Acetaminophen poisoning and toxicity. *Pediatrics* 1975, 55:871–6.)

In acute salicylate poisoning the *Done nomogram* is utilized to guide therapy. It is depicted in Figure 15–2:

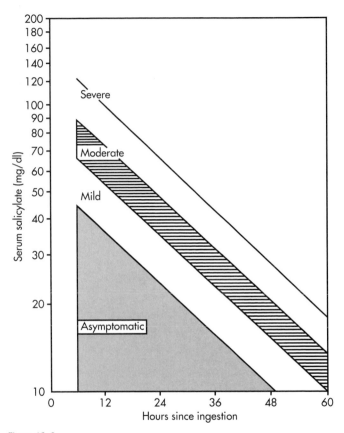

Figure 15–2.
Done nomogram for salicylate poisoning. Note that this nomogram is not accurate for chronic ingestions. (From Done AK: Salicylate intoxication significance of measurements of salicylate in blood in cases of acute ingestion. *Pediatrics* 1960; 26:800–7.)

For any poisoning it is recommended to notify the nearest *poison control center*. Telephone numbers for some of these centers are listed in Table 15–2:

Table 15–2. Telephone numbers of some of the U.S. regional poison control centers

State	City	800 number (in-state only)	Telephone number
Alabama	Birmingham	(800) 292-6678	(205) 939-9201
	Tuscaloosa	(800) 462-0800	(205) 345-0600
Arizona	Phoenix		(602) 253-3334
	Tucson	(800) 362-0101	(602) 626-6016
California	Fresno	(800) 346-5922	(209) 445-1222
	Los Angeles	(800) 825-2722	(213) 484-5151
	Sacramento	(800) 342-9293	(916) 453-3692
	San Diego	(800) 876-4766	(619) 543-6000
	San Francisco	(800) 523-2222	(415) 476-6600
Colorado	Denver	(800) 332-3073	(303) 629-1123
District of Columbia	Washington		(202) 625-3333
Florida	Tampa	(800) 282-3171	(813) 253-4444
Georgia	Atlanta	(800) 282-5846	(404) 589-4400
Kentucky	Louisville	(800) 722-5725	(502) 589-8222
Maryland	Baltimore	(800) 492-2414	(410) 528-7701
Massachusetts	Boston	(800) 682-9211	(617) 232-2120
Michigan	Detroit	(800) 462-6642	(313) 745-5711
	Grand Rapids	(800) 632-2727	(616) 774-7851
Minnesota	Minneapolis		(612) 347-3141
	St. Paul	(800) 222-1222	(612) 221-2113
Missouri	St. Louis	(800) 392-9111	(314) 772-5200
Montana		(800) 332-3073	
Nebraska	Omaha	(800) 642-9999	(402) 390-5400
New Jersey	Newark	(800) 962-1253	(201) 923-0764
New Mexico	Albuquerque	(800) 432-6866	(505) 843-2551
New York	New York City		(212) 340-4494
Ohio	Cincinnati	(800) 872-5111	(513) 558-5111
	Columbus	(800) 682-7625	(614) 228-1323
Oregon	Portland	(800) 452-7165	(503) 279-8968
Pennsylvania	Pittsburgh		(412) 681-6669
	Philadelphia		(215) 386-2100
Rhode Island	Providence		(401) 277-5727
Texas	Austin		(512) 478-4490
	Dallas	(800) 441-0040	(214) 590-5000
	Galveston		(409) 765-9728
	Houston	(800) 392-8548	(713) 654-1701
Utah	Salt Lake City	(800) 456-7707	(801) 581-2151
West Virginia	Charleston	(800) 642-3625	(304) 348-4211
Wyoming		(800) 332-3073	

Trauma

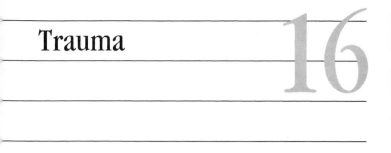

Trauma causes many intensive care unit admissions around the world, and a number of formulas, scores, and indices are available for the assessment and management of these patients.

1. **Hemorrhage:** In order to assess the intravascular volume resuscitation needed in a trauma patient, *normal blood volumes* (according to age) need to be known (Table 16–1).

Table 16–1. Normal blood volumes according to age

Normal blood volumes by age	
Newborn	85 mL/Kg
Infant	80 mL/Kg
Child	75 mL/Kg
Adult	70 mL/Kg

The *severity of hemorrhage* in a trauma patient can be classified as follows (Table 16–2):

Table 16–2. Classification of severity of hemorrhage in trauma patients

Severity of hemorrhage	Blood pressure (mm Hg)	Blood loss (ml)	Plasma volume (ml)
Normal	120/80	—	5000
Class I	120/80	<750	4600
Class II	115/80	1000–1250	3800
Class III	90/70	1500–1800	3200
Class IV	60/40	2000–2500	2500

To estimate how much whole blood or packed red blood cells (PRBC) must be administered to change the hematocrit percentage to a desired amount in a trauma patient, the following formula can be utilized:

Transfusion required (mL) = Desired change in Hct × Kg × factor

where Hct = hematocrit; factor = varies with the volume of blood per body weight (adults and children > 2 years, a factor of 1 will achieve a Hct of 70 percent using PRBC and 1.75 to achieve a Hct of 40 percent using whole blood).

2. Burns: Please refer also to Chapter 3.

Several formulas can be used to guide initial fluid resuscitation after burn injuries. Below are the most common in clinical practice. In all these formulas, 50 percent of the calculated volume is given during the first 8 hours, 25 percent of the calculated volume is given during the second 8 hours, and 25 percent of the calculated volume is given during the third 8 hours.

The *Evans formula* can be calculated as:

Evans formula = 1 mL crystalloid/Kg/% burn/24 h
1 mL colloid/Kg/% burn/24 h
2000 mL D_5W/24 h

The *Brooke formula* and the *modified Brooke formula* are calculated as:

Brooke formula = 1.5 mL crystalloid/Kg/% burn/24 h
0.5 mL colloid/Kg/% burn/24 h
2000 mL D_5W/24 h

Modified formula = 2 mL Ringer's lactate/Kg/% burn/24 h

The *Parkland formula* is calculated as:

Parkland formula = 4 mL crystalloid/Kg/% burn/24 h

In addition to these formulas, the evaporative water losses in patients with burns need to be calculated and those losses replaced. *Evaporative water loss* (EWL) is calculated as:

EWL (mL/h) = (25 + % BSA burned) × BSA

3. Trauma scoring systems: There are several systems in use throughout the world. Of them, the *abbreviated injury scale* (AIS) is often used (Table 16–3).

Table 16–3. The abbreviated injury scale

AIS score	Injury severity
1	Minor
2	Moderate
3	Serious, non-life-threatening
4	Severe, life-threatening
5	Critical
6	Maximal (correlates with death)

The *trauma score* (TS) is another commonly utilized system and is depicted below (Table 16–4).

Table 16–4. The trauma score

Variable	Measurements	Score
Respiratory rate (bpm)	10–24	4
	25–35	3
	>35	2
	<10	1
	0	0
Respiratory effort	Shallow	1
	Retractions	0
Systolic blood pressure (mm Hg)	>90	4
	70–90	3
	50–69	2
	<50	1
	0	0
Capillary refill	Normal	2
	Delayed	1
	Absent	0
Glasgow coma scale	14–15	5
	11–13	4
	8–10	3
	5–7	2
	3–4	1

The *revised trauma score* (RTS) eliminates the assessment of capillary refill and respiratory effort and is calculated as:

$$\text{RTS} = 0.9368\ \text{GCS} + 0.7326\ \text{SBP} + 0.2908\ \text{RR coded values} \times \text{Revised score coefficient}$$

where GCS = Glasgow coma scale; SBP = systolic blood pressure; RR = respiratory rate.

For children and infants, the *pediatric trauma score* is utilized (Table 16–5).

Table 16–5. The pediatric trauma score

Variable	+2	+1	−1
Weight (lb)	>20	10–20	<10
Airway	Normal	Maintained	Nonmaintained
Systolic BP (mm Hg)	>90	50–90	<50
CNS function	Awake	Obtunded	Coma
Open wound	None	Minor	Major
Skeletal trauma	None	Closed	Open or multiple

4. **Neurologic trauma:** Within the primary survey an early neurologic trauma evaluation can be accomplished using the *AVPU method:*

> A = *a*lert
> V = responds to *v*erbal stimulation
> P = responds to *p*ainful stimulation
> U = *u*nresponsive

The *Glasgow coma scale* is another frequently utilized method of assessment of the neurologic status of the trauma patient (Table 16–6).

Table 16–6. Glasgow coma scale

Variable	Score
Eye opening	
Spontaneous	4
To verbal command	3
To pain	2
None	1
Best motor response	
Obeys verbal commands	6
Localizes painful stimuli	5
Flexion-withdrawal from painful stimuli	4
Decorticate (flexion) response to painful stimulation	3
Decerebrate (extension) response to painful stimulation	2
None	1
Best verbal response	
Oriented conversation	5
Disoriented conversation	4
Inappropriate words	3
Incomprehensible sounds	2
None	1

In those patients with severe head injuries and during intracranial pressure monitoring, *cerebral perfusion pressure* (CPP) is commonly utilized in management:

$$CPP = MAP - ICP$$

where MAP = mean arterial blood pressure; ICP = intracranial pressure.

Another useful formula in neurologic trauma is that of the calculation of the *pressure-volume index* (PVI), which is defined as the volume (in mL) necessary to raise the cerebrospinal fluid (CSF) pressure by a factor of 10:

$$PVI = \frac{\Delta V}{\log_{10}(Pp/P_0)}$$

where ΔV = volume change in the lateral ventricle using a ventricular cannula; P_0 = initial ICP; Pp = peak ICP.

17

Common
Laboratory
Values

The most common laboratory values used in the assessment of critically ill patients are presented in this chapter. They have been organized in alphabetical order and according to biologic source where: (P) represents plasma; (B) blood; (S) serum; (U) urine; (CSF) cerebrospinal fluid; (RBCs) red blood cells; and (WBCs) white blood cells. These values are not intended to be definitive, since normal ranges vary from hospital to hospital. Both traditional units and *système international (SI)* units are presented.

α1-Antitrypsin S
150–350 mg/dL (dual report) (*SI*: 1.5–3.5 g/L)

17-Ketogenic steroids (as dehydroepiandrosterone) (U)
Female: 7–12 mg/24 h (*SI*: 25–40 μmol/d)
Male: 9–17 mg/24 h (*SI*: 30–60 μmol/d)

17-Ketosteroids (as dehydroepiandrosterone) (U)
Female: 6–17 mg/24 h (*SI*: 20–60 μmol/d)
Male: 6–20 mg/24 h (*SI*: 20–70 μmol/d)

Alanine aminotransferase (ALT) (S)
0–35 (35°C) Units/L (*SI*: 0–35 U/L)

Albumin (S)
4.0–6.0 g/dL (*SI*: 40–60 g/L)

Ammonia (P)
As ammonia (NH_3): 10–80 μg/dL (dual report) (*SI*: 5–50 μmol/L)
As ammonium (NH_4): 10–85 μg/dL (dual report) (*SI*: 5–50 μmol/L)
As nitrogen (N): 10–65 μg/dL (dual report) (*SI*: 5–50 μmol/L)

Amylase (S):
0–130 (37°C) Units/L (*SI*: 0–130 U/L)
50–150 Somogyi units/dL (*SI*: 100–300 U/L)

Aspartate aminotransferase (AST) (S)
0–35 (37°C) Units/L (*SI:* 0–35 U/L)

Bilirubin (S)
Total: 0.1–1.0 mg/dL (dual report) (*SI*: 2–18 μmol/L)
Conjugated: 0–0.2 mg/dL (dual report) (*SI*: 0–4 μmol/L)

Calcium (S)
Male: 8.8–10.3 mg/dL (dual report) (*SI*: 2.20–2.58 mmol/L)
Female: <50 years 8.8–10.3 mg/dL (dual report) (*SI*: 2.20–2.58 mmol/L)

Calcium, normal diet (U)
<250 mg/24 h (*SI*: <6.2 mmol/d)

Carbon dioxide content (CO_2 + HCO_3) (B,P,S)
22–28 mEq/L (*SI*: 22–28 mmol/L)

Chloride (S)
95–105 mEq/L (*SI*: 95–105 mmol/L)

Cholesterol esters, as a fraction of total cholesterol (P)
60%–75% (*SI*: 0.60–0.75)

Complement, C3 (S)
70–160 mg/dL (*SI*: 0.7–1.6 g/L)

Copper (S)
70–140 μg/dL (*SI*: 11.0–22.0 μmol/L)

Cholesterol (P)
<200 mg/dL (dual report) (*SI*: <5.20 mmol/L)

Copper (U)
<40 μg/24 h (*SI*: <0.6 μmol/d)

Corticotropin (ACTH) (P)
20–100 pg/mL (*SI*: 4–22 pmol/L)

Creatine kinase (CK) (S)
0–130 (37°C) Units/L (*SI*: 0–130 U/L)

Creatine kinase isoenzymes, MB fraction (S)
>5% in myocardial infarction (*SI*: >0.05)

Creatine (U)
Male: 0–40 mg/24 h (*SI*: 0–300 μmol/d)
Female: 0–80 mg/24 h (*SI*: 0–600 μmol/d)

Creatine (S)
  Male: 0.17–0.50 mg/dL (*SI*: 10–40 μmol/L)
  Female: 0.35–0.93 mg/dL (*SI*: 30–70 μmol/L)

Creatinine (U)
  Variable g/24 h (Dual report) (*SI*: variable mmol/d)

Creatinine (S)
  0.6–1.2 mg/dL (dual report) (*SI*: 50–110 μmol/L)

Creatinine clearance (S,U)
  75–125 mL/min (dual report) (*SI*: 1.24–2.08 mL/s)

Cystine (U)
  10–100 mg/24 hr (*SI*: 40–420 μmol/d)

Dehydroepiandrosterone (U)
  Female: 0.2–1.8 mg/24 h (*SI*: 1–6 μmol/d)
  Male: 0.2–2.0 mg/24 h (*SI*: 1–7 μmol/d)

Digoxin, therapeutic (P)
  0.5–2.2 ng/mL (dual report) (*SI*: 0.6–2.8 mmol/L)
  0.5–2.2 μg/L (dual report) (*SI*: 0.6–2.8 mmol/L)

Erythrocyte sedimentation rate (B)
  Female: 0–30 mm/h (*SI*: 0–30 mm/h)
  Male: 0–20 mm/h (*SI*: 0–20 mm/h)

Estradiol, male > 18 y (S)
  15–40 pg/mL (dual report) (*SI*: 55–150 pmol/L)

Ethyl alcohol (P)
  <100 mg/dL (*SI*: <22 mmol/L)

Etiocholanolone
  Female: 0.8–4.0 mg/24 h (*SI*: 2–14 μmol/d)
  Male: 1.4–5.0 mg/14 h (*SI*: 4–17 μmol/d)

Testosterone (P)
  Female: <0.6 ng/mL (dual report) (*SI*: <2.0 nmol/L)
  Male: 4.0–8.0 ng/mL (dual report) (*SI*: 14.0–28.0 nmol/L)

Fibrinogen (P)
  200–4300 mg/dL (*SI*: 2.0–4.0 g/L)

Follicle-stimulating hormone (FSH) (P)
  Female: 2.0–15.0 mIU/mL (*SI*: 2–15 IU/L)
  Peak production: 20–50 mIU/mL (*SI*: 20–50 IU/L)
  Male: 1.0–10.0 mIU/mL (*SI*: 1–10 IU/L)

Follicle-stimulating hormone (FSH) (U)
Follicular phase: 2–15 IU/24 h (*SI*: 2–15 IU/d)
Midcycle: 8–40 IU/24 h (*SI*: 8–40 IU/d)
Luteal phase: 2–10 IU/24 h (*SI*: 2–10 IU/d)
Menopausal women: 35–100 IU/24 h (*SI*: 35–100 IU/d)
Male: 2–15 IU/24 hr (*SI*: 2–15 IU/d)

Gamma-glutamyltransferase (GGT) (S)
0–30 (30°C) Units/L (*SI*: 0–30 U/L)

Glucose (P)
70–110 mg/dL (dual report) (*SI*: 3.9–6.1 mmol/L)

Hematocrit (B)
Female: 33%–43% (*SI*: 0.33–0.43)
Male: 39%–49% (*SI*: 0.39–0.49)

Hemoglobin (B)
Male: 14.0–18.0 g/dL (*SI*: 140–180 g/L)
Female: 11.5–15.5 g/dL (*SI*: 115–155 g/L)

Hemoglobin (B)
Female: 12.0–15.0 g/dL (*SI*: 120–150 g/L)
Male: 13.6–17.2 g/dL (*SI*: 136–172 g/L)

Immunoglobulins (S)
IgG: 500–1200 mg/dL (*SI*: 5.00–12.00 g/L)
IgA: 50–350 mg/dL (*SI*: 0.50–3.50 g/L)
IgM: 30–230 mg/dL (*SI*: 0.30–2.30 g/L)
IgD: <6 mg/dL (*SI*: <60 mg/L)
IgE:
0–3 y: 0.5–1.0 U/ml (*SI*: 1–24 μg/L)
3–80 y: 5–100 U/ml (*SI*: 12–240 μg/L)

Iron (S)
Male: 80–180 μg/dL (dual report) (*SI*: 14–32 μmol/L)
Female: 60–160 μg/dL (dual report) (*SI*: 11–29 μmol/L)

Iron-binding capacity (S)
250–460 μg/dL (dual report) (*SI*: 45–82 μmol/L)

Ketosteroid fractions (U)
Androsterone
Female: 0.5–3.0 mg/24 h (*SI*: 1–10 μmol/d)
Male: 2.0–5.0 mg/24 h (*SI*: 7–17 μmol/d)

Lactate dehydrogenase (S)
50–150 (37°C) Units/L (*SI*: 50–150 U/L)

Lactate dehydrogenase isoenzymes (S)
   LD₁: 15%–40% (*SI*: 0.15–0.40)
   LD₂: 20%–45% (*SI*: 0.20–0.45)
   LD₃: 15%–30% (*SI*: 0.15–0.30)
   LD₄ and LD₅: 5%–20% (*SI*: 0.05–0.20)
   LD₁: 10–60 Units/L (*SI*: 10–60 U/L)
   LD₂: 20–70 Units/L (*SI*: 20–70 U/L)
   LD₃: 10–45 Units/L (*SI*: 10–45 U/L)
   LD₄ and LD₅: 5–30 Units/L (*SI*: 5–30 U/L)

Lead, toxic (B)
   >60 μg/dL (dual report) (*SI*: >2.90 μmol/L)

Lead, toxic (U)
   >80 μg/24 h (dual report) (*SI*: >0.40 μmol/d)

Lipids, total (P)
   400–850 mg/dL (dual report) (*SI*: 4.0–8.5 g/L)

Lipoproteins (P)
   Low-density (LDL), as cholesterol: 50–190 mg/dL (dual report) (*SI*: 1.30–4.90 mmol/L)
   High-density (HDL), as cholesterol:
      Male: 30–70 mg/dL (dual report) (*SI*: 0.80–1.80 mmol/L)
      Female: 30–90 mg/dL (dual report) (*SI*: 0.80–2.35 mmol/L)

Magnesium (S)
   1.8–3.0 mg/dL (dual report) (*SI*: 0.80–1.20 mmol/L)

Mean corpuscular hemoglobin concentration (B)
   Mass concentration: 33–37 g/dL (*SI*: 330–370 g/L)
   Substance concentration (Hb[Fe]): 33–37 g/dL (*SI*: 20–23 mmol/L)

Mean corpuscular hemoglobin (B)
   Mass concentration: 27–33 pg (*SI*: 27–33 pg)
   Substance concentration (Hb[Fe]): 27–33 pg (*SI*: 1.68–2.05 fmol)

Mean corpuscular volume (B)
   Erythrocyte volume: 76–100 cu μm (*SI*: 76–100 fL)

Phenytoin, therapeutic (P)
   10–20 mg/L (*SI*: 40–80 μmol/L)

Phosphatase, acid (prostatic) (P)
   0–3 King-Armstrong Units/dL (*SI*: 0–5.5 U/L)

Phosphatase, alkaline (S)
   30–120 Units/L (*SI*: 30–120 U/L)

Phosphate (as phosphorus) (S)
2.5–5.0 mg/dL (dual report) (*SI*: 0.80–1.60 mmol/L)

Platelets (B)
150–450 10^3/cu mm (*SI*: 150–450 10^9/L)

Potassium (S)
3.5–5.0 mEq/L (*SI*: 3.5–5.0 mmol/L)

Progesterone (P)
Follicular phase: <2 ng/mL (*SI*: <6 nmol/L)
Luteal phase: 2–20 ng/mL (*SI*: 6–64 nmol/L)

Protein, total (U)
<150 mg/24 h (*SI*: <0.15 g/d)

Protein, total (S)
6–8 g/dL (*SI*: 60–80 g/L)

Protein, total (CSF)
<40 mg/dL (*SI*: <0.40 g/L)

Red blood cell count (erythrocytes) (B)
Female: 3.5–5.0 10^6/cu mm (*SI*: 3.5–5.0 10^{12}/L)
Male: 4.3–5.9 10^6/cu mm (*SI*: 4.3–5.1 10^{12}/L)

Red blood cell count (CSF)
0/cu mm (*SI*: 0 10^6/L)

Reticulocyte count (adult) (B)
10,000–75,000/cu mm (dual report) (*SI*: 10–75 × 10^6/L)
Number fraction: 1–24 0/00 (No. per 1000 erythrocytes) (*SI*: 1–24 10^{-3})
        0.1%–2.4% (*SI*: 1–24 10^{-3})

Sodium ion (S)
135–147 mEq/L (*SI*: 135–147 mmol/L)

Sodium (S)
135–147 mEq/L (*SI*: 135–147 mmol/L)

Sodium ion (U)
Diet-dependent mEq/24 h (*SI*: 5–25 mmol/d)

Steroids (U)
Hydroxycorticosteroids (as cortisol)
Female: 2–8 mg/24 h (*SI*: 5–25 μmol/d)
Male: 3–10 mg/24 h (*SI*: 10–30 μmol/d)

Thyroxine (T_4) (S)
4–11 μg/dL (dual report) (*SI*: 51–142 nmol/L)

Thyroxine, free (S)
0.8–2.8 ng/dL (dual report) (*SI*: 10–36 pmol/L)

Thyroxine-binding globulin (TBG) (S)
12–28 μg/dL (dual report) (*SI*: 150–360 nmol/L)

Triiodothyronine (T_3) (S)
75–220 ng/dL (*SI*: 1.2–3.4 nmol/L)

Urate (as uric acid) (S)
2.0–7.0 mg/dL (*SI*: 120–140 μmol/L)

Urate (as uric acid) (U)
Diet-dependent g/24 h (*SI*: diet-dependent mmol/d)

Urea nitrogen (S)
8–18 mg/dL (dual report) (*SI*: 3.0–6.5 mmol/L of urea)

Urea nitrogen (U)
12–20 g/24 h (dual report) (*SI*: 430–700 mmol/d of urea)

Urobilinogen (U)
0–4.0 mg/24 h (*SI*: 0.0–6.8 μmol/d)

White blood cell count (CSF)
0–5/cu mm (*SI*: 0–5 10^6/L)

White blood cell count (B)
3200–9800/cu mm (*SI*: 3.2–9.8 × 10^9/L)

Zinc (S)
75–120 μg/dL (*SI*: 11.5–18.5 μmol/L)

Zinc (U)
150-1200 μg/24 h (*SI*: 2.3–18.3 μmol/d)

Appendix A
Medical Record
Abbreviations

a arterial

(a-A)CO₂ arterial to alveolar gradient for partial pressure of carbon dioxide

(A-a)DO₂ alveolar to arterial gradient for partial pressure of oxygen

Aa alveolar/arterial

A₂ aortic second sound

a̅a̅ of each

AB apical beat

ABC airway, breathing, and circulation

abd abdomen

ABG arterial blood gas

abn abnormal

ABVD doxorubicin (Adriamycin), bleomycin, vinblastine, decarbazine (DTIC)

ac before meals

A/C assist control

ACE angiotensin converting enzyme, adrenocortical extract

acet acetone

aCL anticardiolipin (antibody)

ACLS advanced cardiac life support

ACT activated clotting time

ACTH adrenocorticotropic hormone

ADA American Diabetic Association, American Dietetic Association

ADH antidiuretic hormone

ADL activities of daily living

ad lib as desired, freely

adm admission

AF atrial fibrillation

AFB acid-fast bacilli

a fib atrial fibrillation

A/G albumin/globulin ratio

AG anion gap

AIDS acquired immune deficiency syndrome

AJ ankle jerk

AKA above-knee amputation

AL arterial line

alb albumin

alk phos alkaline phosphatase

ALL acute lymphoblastic leukemia

ALS amyotrophic lateral sclerosis

ALT alanine aminotransferase

AM morning

AMA against medical advice

AMI acute myocardial infarction

AML acute myelogenous leukemia

amp ampule

AMP adenosine monophosphate

amt amount

amy amylase

ANA antinuclear antibodies

ANCA antineutrophil cytoplasmic antibody

ANLL acute nonlymphocytic leukemia

AODM adult-onset diabetes mellitus

AOP aortic pressure

A&P auscultation and percussion

AP anteroposterior

APAG antipseudomonal aminoglycosidic penicillin

appt appointment

APSAC anisoylated plasminogen/streptokinase activator complex

APTT activated partial thromboplastin time

APUD   amine precursor uptake decar-
boxylase

aq   water

AR   aortic regurgitation

ARC   AIDS-related complex

ARDS   acute respiratory distress syndrome, adult respiratory dis-
tress syndrome

ARF   acute renal failure

ART   assessment, review, and treatment

AS   atriosystolic, aortic stenosis

asa   aspirin

A.S.A.   American Society of Anesthe-
siologists

ASH   asymmetric septal hypertrophy

ASHD   arteriosclerotic heart disease

ASLO   anti-streptolysin O

AST   aspartate aminotransferase

ATC   around the clock

ATG   antithymocyte globulin

ATN   acute tubular necrosis

AV   arteriovenous, atrioventricular

AVM   arteriovenous malformation

AVP   arginine vasopressin

AZT   zidovudine

B   black

ba   barium

BACOD   bleomycin, doxorubicin
(Adriamycin), cyclophosphamide vincristine (Oncovin),
dexamethasone

BACOP   bleomycin, doxorubicin
(Adriamycin), cyclophosphamide, vincristine (Oncovin),
prednisone

BAL   British anti-Lewisite (dimercaprol)

BBB   bundle-branch block

BC   blood culture

BCG   bacillus Calmette-Guérin

BCNU   carmustine

BCP   birth control pill

BE   barium enema

BEE   basal energy expenditure

bid   two times a day

bilat   bilateral

bili   bilirubin

BiPAP   bi-level positive airway pressure

BKA   below-knee amputation

Bl s   blood sugar

BM   bowel movement

BMR   basal metabolic rate

BP   blood pressure

BPH   benign prostatic hypertrophy

bpm   beats per minute

BR   bed rest

BRP   bathroom privileges

BS or bs   breath sounds, blood sugar,
bowel sounds

BSA   body surface area

BSO   bilateral salpingo-oophorectomy

BTL   bilateral tubal ligation

BUN   blood urea nitrogen

BW   body weight

Bx   biopsy

c̄   with

C   centigrade

C3 to C6   protein components of complement system

Ca   cancer

Ca^{+2}   calcium

(Ca-Cv̄O$_2$)   arterial to mixed venous difference in blood oxygen
concentration

C/A   Clinitest and acetone

CAB   coronary artery bypass

CABG   coronary artery bypass graft

CAD   coronary artery disease

CAF   cyclophosphamide, doxorubicin
(Adriamycin), 5-fluorouracil

cal   calorie

CaO$_2$ arterial oxygen content

cap   capsule

CAT   computerized axial tomography

cath   catheterization

CAV   cyclophosphamide, doxorubicin
(Adriamycin), vincristine

CBC   complete blood cell count

CBD   common bile duct

cc   cubic centimeter

CC   chief complaint

CCr   creatine clearance

CCU   coronary care unit

CD4   helper-inducer T cells

CD8   suppressor-cytotoxic T cell

Cdyn   dynamic compliance of the lung

CEA   carcinoembryonic antigen

CF   complement fixation, conversion
factor

CGL   chronic granulocytic (myelogenous) leukemia

CHD congenital heart disease
CHF congestive heart failure
CHO carbohydrate
CHOP cyclophosphamide, doxorubicin, vincristine (Oncovin), prednisone
CI cardiac index
CIE counterimmunoelectrophoresis
CK creatine kinase
CK-MB creatine kinase, myocardial band
cl clear
Cl⁻ chloride
CLL chronic lymphocytic leukemia
cm centimeter
CM costal margin
CMF cyclophosphamide, methotrexate, 5-fluorouracil
CML chronic myelogenous leukemia
CMV cytomegalovirus, controlled mechanical ventilation
CNS central nervous system
CO cardiac output, carbon monoxide
c/o complains of
CO₂ carbon dioxide
CoA coenzyme A
COMLA cyclophosphamide, vincristine (Oncovin), methotrexate, leucovorin, cytosine araabinoside
conc concentrate
COPD chronic obstructive pulmonary disease
CPAP continuous positive airway pressure
CPK creatine phosphokinase
CPR cardiopulmonary resuscitation
Cr creatinine
CR cardiorespiratory
CRH corticotropin releasing hormone
C/S culture and sensitivity
CSF cerebrospinal fluid
C/sec cesarean section
Cst static compliance of the lung
CT computed tomography
Cu copper
CV cardiovascular
cva costovertebral angle
CVA cerebrovascular accident
CV̄O₂ mixed venous oxygen content

CVP central venous pressure
CXR chest X-ray
cysto cystoscopy
D&C dilation and curettage
D/C discontinue
D&S dilation and suction
DAT diet as tolerated
DBIL direct bilirubin
DCF 2′ deoxycoformycin
DDAVP desmopressin
ddI dideoxyinosine
DFA direct fluorescent antibody
DGI disseminated gonococcal infection
DHPG ganciclovir
Dial dialysis
DIC disseminated intravascular coagulation
dil dilute
DIP distal interphalangeal, desquamative interstitial pneumonitis
DKA diabetic ketoacidosis
DL_{CO} diffusing capacity of lung for carbon monoxide
dl deciliter
DLE drug-related lupus erythematosus
DM diabetes mellitus
DNA deoxyribonucleic acid
DOA dead on arrival
ḊO₂ oxygen delivery
ḊO₂(I) oxygen delivery index
DP dorsalis pedis
DPT diphtheria, pertussis, tetanus
DR delivery room
ds double strand
DSD dry sterile dressing
DTIC dacarbazine
DTR deep tendon reflex
DTs delirium tremens
DU duodenal ulcer
DUB dysfunctional uterine bleeding
DVT deep venous thrombosis
D₅W dextrose (5%) in water
Dx diagnosis
EBL estimated blood loss
EBV Epstein-Barr virus
ECF extended care facility, extracellular fluid
ECG electrocardiogram
ECM erythema chronicum migrans
ED emergency department

EDTA   ethylene diamine tetraacetate
EEG   electroencephalogram
EENT   eyes, ears, nose, and throat
EF   ejection fraction
EIA   electroimmunoassay
EKG   electrocardiogram
elect   electrolyte
ELISA   enzyme-linked immunoassay
elix   elixir
EMD   electromechanical dissociation
EMG   electromyogram
ENT   ear, nose, and throat
EOM   extraocular movements
EPO   erythropoietin
EPS   extrapyramidal symptoms
ER   emergency room, estrogen receptor
ERCP   endoscopic retrograde cholangi-
opancreatography
ERS   evacuation retained secundines
ERV   expiratory reserve volume
ESR   erythrocyte sedimentation rate
ESRD   end-stage renal disease
EST, ECT   electroshock therapy, elec-
troconvulsive therapy
et al   and others
EUA   examination under anesthesia
ext   extract, extremities
f   respiratory rate
F   Fahrenheit
FABM3   acute promyelocytic leukemia
FBS   fasting blood sugar
FDP   fibrin degradation products
Fe   iron
FE   fractional excretion
FEV   forced expiratory volume
FF   force fluids
FFP   fresh frozen plasma
FH   family history
FHM   fetal heart monitor
FHR   fetal heart rate
FIo$_2$ fraction of inspired oxygen
fl   fluid, femtoliter
fL   femtoliter
FMF   familial Mediterranean fever
FNA   fine needle aspiration
FRC   functional residual capacity
FS   frozen section
FSH   follicle stimulating hormone
FTA-ABS   fluorescent treponemal anti-
body absorbed

FTI   free thyroxine index
5-FU   5-fluorouracil
FUO   fever of undetermined origin
FVC   forced vital capacity
fx   fracture
g   gram
Ga   gallium
GA   general anesthesia
GB   gallbladder
Gc   gonococcus
GERD   gastroesophageal reflux disease
GFR   glomerular filtration rate
GGT   γ-glutamyltransferase
GGTP   γ-glutamyltranspeptidase
GI   gastrointestinal
GIP   gastric inhibitory polypeptide
GITS   gastrointestinal therapeutic
system
glu   glucose
GN   glomerulonephritis
G$_6$PD   glucose-6-phosphate dehydro-
genase
gr   grain
GSW   gun shot wound
gtt   drop
GTT   glucose tolerance test
GU   genitourinary
GVHD   graft versus host disease
G/W   enema glycerine and water enema
Gyn   gynecology
H$_2$ histamine$_2$
H/A   headache
HA   hyperalimentation
HAV   hepatitis A virus
Hb   hemoglobin
HB$_c$Ag   hepatitis B core antigen
HB$_s$Ag   hepatitis B surface antigen
HBIG   hepatitis B immune globulin
HBP   high blood pressure
HBV   hepatitis B virus
HCO$_3^-$ bicarbonate
hct   hematocrit
HCV   hepatitis C virus
HD   hospital discharge
HDL   high-density lipoprotein
HDV   hepatitis D virus
HEENT   head, eyes, ears, nose, and
throat
Hg   hemoglobin
H/H   hemoglobin/hematocrit

5-HIAA   5-hydroxyindoleacetic acid
HIV   human immunodeficiency virus
H&L   heart and lungs
HLA   human leukocyte antigen
HMG-CoA   3-hydroxy-3-methylglutaryl coenzyme A
HNP   herniated nucleus pulposus
H₂O   water
H₂O₂   hydrogen peroxide
HOCM   hypertrophic obstructive cardiomyopathy
HORF   high-output renal failure
H&P   history and physical exam
HPI   history of present illness
HR   heart rate
HRS   hepatorenal syndrome
hs   hour of sleep (at bedtime)
HSV   herpes simplex virus
ht   height
HTN   hypertension
hx   history
I&D   incision and drainage
IABP   intraaortic balloon pump
IBC   iron-binding capacity
IBD   inflammatory bowel disease
IBS   irritable bowel syndrome
IC   inspiratory capacity
ICF   intracellular fluid
ICP   intracranial pressure
ICU   intensive care unit
ID   intradermal
IDDM   insulin-dependent diabetes mellitus
IFA   immunofluorescent assay
Ig   immunoglobulin
IHSS   idiopathic hypertrophic subaortic stenosis
ILD   interstitial lung disease
IM   intramuscular
Imp   impression
IMV   intermittent mandatory ventilation
inf   infusion
inh   inhalation
inj   injection
I&O   intake and output
IOP   intraocular pressure
IPG   impedance plethysmography
iPLP   parathyroid hormone-like protein by radioimmunoassay

IPPB   intermittent positive pressure breathing
iPTH   parathyroid hormone by radioimmunoassay
IQ   intelligence quotient
ISG   immune serum globulin
ITP   idiopathic thrombocytopenic purpura
IUD   intrauterine device
IV   intravenous
IVC   inferior vena cava
IVP   intravenous pyelogram
J   joule
JG   juxtaglomerular
JVD   jugular venous distention
JVP   jugular vein pulse
kat   katal (mole/sec)
K⁺   potassium
KJ   knee jerk
Kg   kilogram
17-KS   17-ketosteroid
KUB   kidney, ureter, and bladder
l   left
L   liters, vascular volume
LA   left atrium
lab   laboratory
lac   laceration
LAD   left axis deviation
LAHB   left anterior hemiblock
lap   laparotomy
LAP   leukocyte alkaline phosphatase
LAV   lymphadenopathy-associated virus (same as HIV)
lb   pound
LBBB   left bundle-branch block
LBP   low back pain
LDH   lactate dehydrogenase
LDL   low density lipoprotein
LES   lower esophageal sphincter
LFT   liver function test
LGV   lymphogranuloma venereum
LH   luteinizing hormone
LHRH   luteinizing hormone-releasing hormone
Li   lithium
Lip   lipid
liq   liquid
LLL   left lower lobe
LLQ   left lower quadrant
LMD   local medical doctor

LMP last menstrual period
LNMP last normal menstrual period
LOC level of consciousness
LP lumbar puncture
LPHB left posterior hemiblock
LSB left sternal border
LSK liver, spleen, and kidney
LUL left upper lobe
LUSB left upper sternal border
LUQ left upper quadrant
LVEDP left ventricular end diastolic pressure
LVH left ventricular hypertrophy
LVSWI left ventricular stroke work index
L & W living and well
m murmur
M midnight, monoclonal
M1 to M7 categories of ANLL
MACE methotrexate, doxorubicin (Adriamycin), cyclophosphamide, epipodophyllotoxin
MAI *Mycobacterium avium intracellulare*
MAO monoamine oxidase
MAP mean arterial pressure
MAT multi-focal atrial tachycardia
max maximum
MB isoenzyme of cardiac origin
MBC minimum bactericidal concentration
MCA middle cerebral artery
MCL midclavicular line
MCP metacarpophalangeal
MCTD mixed connective tissue disease
MCV mean cell volume
med medication
MED medical
MEN multiple endocrine neoplasia
mEq milliequivalent
MERSA methicillin-resistant *Staphylococcus aureus*
mets metastases
MF maturation factor
mg milligram
Mg^{2+} magnesium
MH malignant hyperthermia
MHTAP microhemagglutination assay for antibody to *Treponema pallidum*

MI myocardial infarction
MIBG meta-iodobenzyl guanidine
MIC minimum inhibitory concentration
min minute
mixt mixture
μkat microkatal (micromole/sec)
ml milliliter
ML malignant lymphoma
μmol micromole
mm millimeter
mM, mmol millimole
mod moderate
MOM milk of magnesia
MOPP mechlorethamine, vincristine (Oncovin), procarbazine, prednisone
mOsm milliosmol
MP metacarpophalangeal
MPGN membrane proliferative glomerulonephritis
MPTP analog of meperidine (used by drug addicts)
MR mitral regurgitation
MRI magnetic resonance imaging
MS mitral stenosis, mental status
MSU monosodium urate
MTC medullary thyroid carcinoma
MTP metatarsophalangeal
MUGA multiple gated (image) acquisition (analysis)
MVA motor vehicle accident
MVP mitral valve prolapse; mitomycin, vinblastine, cisplatin (Platinol)
MVV maximum voluntary ventilation
N normal
NA not applicable
Na^+ sodium
$NaHCO_3$ sodium bicarbonate
NAPA N-acetyl-procainamide, N-acetyl-paraaminophenol
NAS no added sodium
NB newborn
NCP nursing care plan
neg negative
NETT nasal endotracheal tube
Neuro neurology
ng nanogram
NG nasogastric
NGU nongonococcal urethritis
NH_3 ammonia

NHL   non-Hodgkin's lymphoma
NIDDM   non–insulin-dependent diabetes mellitus
NKA   no known allergy
nkat   nanokatal (nanomole/sec)
NKDA   no known drug allergies
NM   neuromuscular
no   number
noc   night, nocturnal
NPH   normal pressure hydrocephalus, neutral protamine Hagedorn (insulin)
NPO   nothing by mouth
NS   normal saline
NSAID   nonsteroidal antiinflammatory drug
NSILA   nonsuppressible insulin-like activity
NSR   normal sinus rhythm
NTG   nitroglycerin
NYHA   New York Heart Association
OA   oral airway
OAF   osteoclast activity factor
OB   obstetrics
OD   overdose; right eye
OETT   oral endotracheal tube
17-OHCS   17-hydroxycorticosteroid
25-OHD   1,25-dihydroxyvitamin D
oint   ointment
OOB   out of bed
OPD   outpatient department
opt   optimum
ophth   ophthalmology
OR   operating room
Oral   oral surgery
Ortho or ortho   orthopedics
OS   left eye
osm   osmolality
OT   occupational therapy
OU   each eye
oz   ounce
p   pulse
$\bar{\text{p}}$ after
P wave   part of the electrocardiographic cycle representing atrial depolarization (stimulation)
P$_2$ pulmonic second sound
Paco$_2$ partial pressure of CO_2 in arterial blood

Pao$_2$ partial pressure of O_2 in arterial blood
P$_A$O$_2$ partial pressure of oxygen in the alveolar gas
P&A   percussion and auscultation
PA   posteroanterior, pulmonary artery
PADP   pulmonary artery diastolic pressure
P$_{ALV}$ alveolar pressure
PAOP   pulmonary artery occlusion pressure (wedge)
Pap   Papanicolaou
PAP   pulmonary artery pressure
para   number of pregnancies
PAS   paraaminosalicylic acid
PASP   pulmonary artery systolic pressure
PAT   paroxysmal atrial tachycardia
PAWP   pulmonary artery wedge pressure
pc   after meals
Pco$_2$ carbon dioxide tension
PCP   *Pneumocystis carinii* pneumonia, phencyclidine
PCWP   pulmonary capillary wedge pressure
PE   physical exam, pulmonary embolism
PEA   pulseless electrical activity
ped   pediatric
PEEP   positive end-expiratory pressure
PEEP$_i$ intrinsic PEEP, autoPEEP
PEFR   peak expiratory flow rate
per   by
PERRLA   pupils equal, round, reactive to light and accommodation
PFT   pulmonary function test
pg   picogram
PGE   prostaglandin E
PH   past history
phos   phosphorus
PHP   pseudohypoparathyroidism
PHR   peak heart rate
PI   present illness
PID   pelvic inflammatory disease
PIP   proximal interphalangeal
PKU   phenylketonuria
PLA   plasminogen activator
PLP   parathyroid hormone-like protein
PM   afternoon

PMI point of maximum impulse
PMN polymorphonuclear leukocyte
PMP previous menstrual period
PM & R physical medicine and rehabilitation
PMR polymyalgia rheumatica
PND paroxysmal nocturnal dyspnea
PNH paroxysmal nocturnal hemoglobinuria
PO by mouth
PO₄ phosphate
postop postoperative
Po₂ oxygen tension
PP postpartum
PPD purified protein derivative
PPNG penicillinase-producing *Neisseria gonorrhoeae*
PR per rectum, pulmonic regurgitation, progesterone receptor
PR interval part of electrocardiographic cycle from onset of atrial depolarization to onset of ventricular depolarization
Pra right atrial pressure
preop preoperative
prep preparation
PROM premature rupture of membranes
prn as needed
PRSP penicillinase-resistant synthetic penicillin
PS pulmonic stenosis
(PS) pressure support
PSGN post-streptococcal glomerulonephritis
psi pounds per square inch
PSVT paroxysmal supraventricular tachycardia
Psych or psych psychiatry
pt patient
PT prothrombin time, physical therapy, posterior tibia
PTA prior to admission
PTC percutaneous transhepatic cholangiography
PTCA percutaneous transluminal coronary angioplasty
Pth pathology
PTH parathormone

PTRA percutaneous transluminal renal angioplasty
PTT partial thromboplastin time
PTU propylthiouracil
PUD peptic ulcer disease
PVC premature ventricular contraction
PVR pulmonary vascular resistance
PVR(I) pulmonary vascular resistance index
PWP pulmonary wedge pressure
PX physical
q every
Q̇ blood flow
qd every day
qh every hour
qhs every bedtime
qid four times a day
qns quantity not sufficient
Q̇O₂ oxygen transport
qod every other day
QRS part of electrocardiographic wave representing ventricular depolarization (stimulation)
qs quantity sufficient
Q̇ₛ shunt blood flow
Q̇ₛ/Q̇ₜ shunt fraction
r right
R respiratory rate (per min), respiratory quotient
RA rheumatoid arthritis, right atrium
RAI radioactive iodine
RAN resident's admission note
RAP right atrial pressure
Raw airway resistance to air flow into the lung
RBBB right bundle branch block
RBC red blood cells
RDS respiratory distress syndrome
RDW red cell distribution width
R&E round and equal
readm readmission
REM rapid eye movement
RF rheumatoid factor
Rh *Rhesus* blood factor
RIA radioimmunoassay
RIND reversible ischemic neurologic deficit
RL Ringer's lactate
RLL right lower lobe
RLQ right lower quadrant

RML   right middle lobe
RN   registered nurse
RNA   ribonucleic acid
R/O   rule out
ROM   range of motion
ROS   review of systems
RPGN   rapidly progressive glomerulo-
     nephritis
RPI   reticulocyte production index
RPR   rapid plasma reagin
rpt   repeat
RQ   respiratory quotient
RR   recovery room
RSR   regular sinus rhythm
rt-PA   recombinant tissue plasminogen
     activator
R/T   related to
rT_3 reverse triiodothyronine
RTA   renal tubular acidosis
RTC   return to clinic
RUL   right upper lobe
RUQ   right upper quadrant
RV   right ventricle, residual volume
RVH   renovascular hypertension, right
     ventricular hypertrophy
Rx   therapy, treatment, prescription
S_1 first heart sound
S_2 second heart sound
S_3 third heart sound
S_4 fourth heart sound
$\bar{s}$ without
S/A   sugar and acetone
SA   sinoatrial
SAH   subarachnoid hemorrhage
Sao$_2$ percent saturation of hemoglobin
     with oxygen in arterial blood
sat   saturated
SB   stillbirth
SBE   subacute bacterial (infective) en-
     docarditis
SBP   spontaneous bacterial peritonitis
SBT   serum bacterial titer
SC   subcutaneous
SCP   standard care plan
SDH   subdural hematoma
SGA   small for gestational age
SGOT   serum glutamic-oxaloacetic trans-
     aminase (aspartate aminotrans-
     ferase, AST)

SGPT   serum glutamic pyruvate trans-
     aminase (alanine aminotransfer-
     ase, ALT)
SI   Système Internationale
SIADH   syndrome of inappropriate se-
     cretion of antidiuretic hormone
SL   sublingual
SLE   systemic lupus erythematosus
SLR   straight leg raising
SMI   suggested minimum increment
SMS   somatostatin
SNF   skilled nursing facility
SO$_2$ oxygen saturation
SOB   short of breath
SOC   state of consciousness
sol   solution
S/P   status post
SQ   subcutaneous
SR   slow release
SRM   spontaneous rupture membranes
$\overline{ss}$ half
S/S   signs and symptoms
SS   Sjögren's syndrome
SSE   soap suds enema
SSKI   saturated solution potassium
     iodide
SSS   sick sinus syndrome
ST   **segment**   part of electrocardio-
     graphic cycle represent-
     ing the beginning of ven-
     tricular repolarization
     (recovery)
stat   immediately
STD   sexually transmitted disease
STS   serologic test for syphilis
subcu, SC   subcutaneous
supp   suppository
Surg   surgery
susp   suspension
SV   stroke volume
SVC   superior vena cava
S$\bar{v}$o$_2$ percent saturation of hemoglobin
     with oxygen in mixed venous
     blood
SVR   systemic vascular resistance
SVT   supraventricular tachycardia
Sx   symptoms
syr   syrup

T wave part of ECG cycle, representing a portion of ventricular repolarization (recovery)

T_3 triiodothyronine

T_4 thyroxine

T & A tonsillectomy and adenoidectomy

tab tablet

TAH total abdominal hysterectomy

TB tuberculosis

TBG thyroxine binding globulin, total blood gases

TBIL total bilirubin

TBNa total body sodium

Tbsp tablespoon

TBW total body water

T/C throat culture

temp temperature

TENS transcutaneous electrical nerve stimulation

Tg thyroglobulin

THBR thyroid hormone-binding ratio

TIA transient ischemic attack

TIBC total iron-binding capacity

tid three times daily

tinc tincture

TLC total lung capacity

TM tympanic membrane

TMP-SMX trimethoprim/sulfamethoxazole

TNM tumor-nodes-metastases

TO telephone order

top topical

TP total protein

tPA tissue plasminogen activator

TPI *Treponema pallidum* immobilization

TPN total parenteral nutrition

TPR temperature, pulse, and respiration

TR tricuspid regurgitation

TRAP tartrate-resistant acid phosphatase

TRF thyrotropin releasing factor

T_3**RIA** triiodothyronine level by radioimmunoassay

T_3**RU** T_3 resin uptake

TRH thyrotropin releasing hormone

TRIG triglycerides

TS tricuspid stenosis

TSAb thyroid stimulating antibodies

TSH thyroid stimulating hormone

tsp teaspoon

TT thrombin time

TTP thrombotic thrombocytopenic purpura, ribothymidine 5′ triphosphate

TTS transdermal therapeutic system

TU tuberculin unit

TUR transurethral resection

TURP transurethral resection prostate

TV tidal volume

Tx therapy

U unit

UA umbilical artery

U/A urinalysis

UGI upper gastrointestinal

ung ointment

U/P urine/plasma ratio (concentration)

URAC uric acid

URI upper respiratory tract infection

USP United States Pharmacopeia

UTI urinary tract infection

UV ultraviolet

$\bar{v}$ mixed venous

V volume

$\dot{V}$ volume of ventilation per minute

V_A alveolar gas volume

vag hyst vaginal hysterectomy

VAMP vincristine, doxorubicin (Adriamycin), methylprednisolone

VAT ventricular activation time

VC vital capacity

$\dot{V}_{co}$ rate of carbon monoxide uptake per min

VD venereal disease

VDRL Venereal Disease Research Laboratories (test for syphilis)

V_D/V_T ratio of dead-space volume to tidal volume

VER visual evoked response

VF ventricular fibrillation

VIP vasoactive intestinal polypeptide

VLDL very low density lipoprotein

VMA vanillylmandelic acid

VPC ventricular premature contraction

VO verbal order

$\dot{V}O_2$ oxygen consumption

$\dot{V}O_2(I)$ oxygen consumption index

V/Q scan ventilation/perfusion scan

VR venous return	**SYMBOLS**
vs visit	**@** at
VS vital signs	**++** moderate amount
VSD ventricular septal defect	**+++** large amount
V$_T$ tidal volume	**0** zero, none
VT/VF ventricular tachycardia/fibrillation	**°** degree
W white	**♀** female
WBC white blood (cell) count	**♂** male
w/c wheel chair	**#** number
WD well developed	**↑** increased
WF white female	**↓** decreased
WHO World Health Organization	**>** greater than
WM white male	**<** less than
WN well nourished	**μ or μm** micron (micrometer)
WNL within normal limits	**″** seconds
WPW Wolff Parkinson White	**′** minute
wt weight	**ø** absence of
y/o years old	**✔** check
X times	**−** negative, absence
ZDV zidovudine	**△** changes
Z-E Zollinger-Ellison (syndrome)	

NOTICE: The science of medicine is constantly evolving. Every attempt has been made by the author and consultants to ensure that this manual includes the latest recommendations from the medical literature. Doses of drugs and treatment recommendations have been carefully reviewed. **However, it is strongly recommended that the reader become completely familiar with the manufacturer's product information when prescribing any of the drugs described in this manual.** This recommendation is especially important with new or infrequently used drugs. As new information becomes available, changes in treatment modalities invariably follow; therefore when choosing a particular treatment, the reader should consider not only the information provided in this manual but also any recently published medical literature on the subject.

Reprinted from Varon J, ed: *Practical Guide to the Care of the Critically Ill Patient.* St. Louis, Mosby–Year Book, Inc., 1994:1–2.

Appendix B
Key Telephone Numbers

This chapter is a listing of the phone numbers of departments and individuals in the hospital who might be needed for immediate consultation.

Department

Admitting	_____
Anesthesia	_____
CCU	_____
ECG	_____
EEG	_____
ER	_____
ICU	_____
MICU	_____
SICU	_____
PICU	_____
NICU	_____
	_____
	_____
	_____
Information	_____
IV Team	_____
Laboratory	_____
Chemistry	_____
Hematology	_____
Microbiology	_____
Other	_____
Medical Records	_____
Nuclear Medicine	_____
Paging	_____
Pathology	_____
Pharmacy	_____
Physical Therapy	_____
Pulmonary Function	_____
Radiology	_____

Recovery Room
PACU
Respiratory Therapy
Security
Social Service
Ultrasonography
Other

Nursing Stations

House Staff

Attending Staff

_____   _____
_____   _____
_____   _____
_____   _____
_____   _____
_____   _____
_____   _____
_____   _____
_____   _____
_____   _____
_____   _____
_____   _____
_____   _____
_____   _____
_____   _____
_____   _____

Other

_____   _____
_____   _____
_____   _____
_____   _____

Index

Notes

Notes

Notes

Notes

Notes

Notes

Notes

Notes

Notes

Notes

Notes